REVIEWS FOR

EAT SLEEP MOVE BREATHE

I love this book! If you asked me to take decades of experience working at the bleeding edge of human athletic performance and boil it to the most essential behaviors for long term, sustainable success, it would be this book! The trick to unlocking our incredibly robust and antifragile natures is to appreciate the way that the keystone behaviors in this book integrate into a cogent whole. Performing these "basics" well for the rest of your life will never get old or go out of style. The principles within these pages are the fundamentals of being a truly savage human.

—Dr. Kelly Starrett, DPT
Coach, Physio, Co-Founder of The Ready State 2x NYT Best Selling Author

***

I found that this book "Eat, Sleep, Move, Breathe" was very well researched and written. The book is easy to read and to follow. I believe this book provides a well-rounded approach to gain and maintain great health.

—Dr. Harold J. Bowersox, D.O., M.B.A., M.S
Author "The Bowersox Protocol for Fibromyalgia and Chronic Fatigue"

***

Eat Sleep Move Breathe is a wonderful introductory guide to living more fully. As basic global health has shifted over the past 50 years due to changes in our work environments, food supply and traditional ways of living, each of the components the authors address is crucial for health and vitality. As experts in this field, the authors use wonderful stories to make the steps to wellness accessible and simple to implement. They cover the most important aspects of health, healing and vitality; spending time with this book and implementing the recommendations will jump you from a wellness novice into a lifestyle deeply rooted in the transformation into health and vitality.

—Dr. Ann Marie Chiasson
Director of Fellowship in Integrative Medicine, Associate Clinical Professor of Medicine, Andrew Weil Center for Integrative Medicine, University of Arizona, Tucson, Arizona

EAT
SLEEP
MOVE
BREATHE

The Beginner's Guide to Living
A Healthy Lifestyle

Lars Thestrup, MD
Jenny Pfleghaar, DO
Connor Martin

Published by KHARIS PUBLISHING, imprint of KHARIS MEDIA LLC.

Copyright © 2020 Lars Thestrup, MD. Jenny Pfleghaar, DO. Connor Martin

ISBN-13: 978-1-946277-78-7
ISBN-10: 1-946277-78-9

Library of Congress Control Number: 2020943682

All KHARIS PUBLISHING products are available at special quantity discounts for bulk purchase for sales promotions, premiums, fund-raising, and educational needs.
For details, contact:

Kharis Media LLC
Tel: 1-479-599-8657
support@kharispublishing.com
www.kharispublishing.com

CONTENTS

INTRODUCTION

Back when humans made buildings from stone, the most important block they quarried was the cornerstone. This was the first stone set in the construction of the building. In fact, all other stones that came after would reference that foundational setting stone. That's what made them so vital. If your cornerstone was true, the building would be true.

When it comes to personal health, there seems to be a lot of shaky ground and a lot of crooked stones, so it's hard to know how to build a strong, healthy foundation. Within this book, we've developed four cornerstones for building a healthy lifestyle: diet, sleep, meditation, and exercise. If we can each get these concepts set as our cornerstones, we can have a stable foundation for structuring our health.

So where did this idea come from?

I have worked in the ER for 15 years. In that time, I've seen many cases of chronic diseases like diabetes, hypertension (HTN), and coronary artery disease. Many of these diseases afflicting my patients would have been preventable if only they had lived a healthier lifestyle.

During this era of pandemics, there's even greater value in being healthy. Eliminating underlying medical conditions could help you have better outcomes, should you fall ill.

Not long ago, I saw a young person in their early twenties in the ER. They were morbidly obese with multiple health problems. I remember them asking me, "Why do I have these problems? Why am I so obese?"

So, I began asking questions about their lifestyle. I found out they ate fast food three times a day. They were sleeping four hours a night. They had no time for themselves. And exercise? Walking to and from their vehicle made them winded. Diet, sleep, meditation, exercise? Apparently, no one had ever told them about the importance of these behaviors. Sure, they had seen books on these topics, but they were too long and dense; they were overwhelming. This lack of basic facts is what gave birth to the concept of a beginner's guide, a quick and easily digestible manual that lays out the cornerstones of a healthy lifestyle.

Part of the beauty of this concept is simplicity. These four cornerstones all rely on each other to create a stable foundation. Without a healthy diet, your exercise performance suffers. Without exercise, your ability to get good, restful sleep is hindered. When you're sleep-deprived, your mental health can be affected. And when you're not thinking straight, you're more likely to make poor decisions with your diet. Each one has a direct impact on the other. So, if we can get each cornerstone concept right, we can have a stronger body and a more stable mind.

We aren't suggesting you have to chisel out all four healthy concepts to be successful. Focusing your energy on just one, even in the most simple and basic way, can have a profound impact on your health. You can improve your life in big ways by committing to a small change in behavior. Take it one day at a time. Gradually ease into the concept that most interests you. Over time you will find yourself eating healthier, sleeping better, focusing on your mental well-being, and even moving and exercising more. It's not a diet or fad and it's not a program to follow. Think of it as a process, a natural progression. Just make yourself these two promises:

1. I will start by making one small change
2. I will not be too hard on myself

After all, as the old adage goes, *Rome wasn't built in a day*, rather it was built one stone at a time. With these four cornerstones of health, you'll be on the way to building a better you. There is only improvement!

EAT

THE CAUSE AND THE CURE

A M was a young woman I saw frequently in the ER where I worked, so frequently in fact, that I probably saw her more often than her primary care doctor.

She was only in her 20s, and as you could guess, she was not in good health. She could carry on daily activities but AM was not enjoying life. She was overweight. Her joints ached. She was plagued with belly pain and chronic yeast infections. With all her health issues and constant ER visits, AM suffered from depression as well. She was tired, and carrying around all that extra weight was not good for her body. She was weary of it all.

On one of her visits, I had to tell her if she kept coming into the ER with chronic abdominal pain, with all the CT scans she was getting, she was going to increase her risk of radiation cancer; it was getting that bad for her.

I tried to help her. We talked about changing her diet, eliminating the pop, chips, and fast food. We talked

1

about keeping a food diary. I wanted AM to log which foods triggered her reflux. Those simple steps, just that realization, was the "Aha" moment for her. Nutrition was the key. Fueling up on the right foods was the answer to her problems.

With a basic switch, like swapping fresh fruit and vegies for processed food, AM could be on a completely different path. It's so simple, yet so many individuals don't focus on this pillar of health. Beyond that, so many people don't even know where to start, or why eating fast food is such a big deal. That's where a little bit of knowledge comes in. A small amount of know-how can have a profound impact. If we know what we're supposed to eat, and the why behind it, there's a greater motivation to change.

I am not sure what happened to AM after our chat because I stopped working at that ER, but I can say she wasn't the first (or the last) patient I would see in the ER with nutrition as the cause and the cure of their disease.

LET'S BEGIN

We have all heard this saying before but is it true: *You are what you eat.* What you put into your body can make a difference in how you look, how you feel, and how you act. Not only is food used for energy, but the correct food can help prevent cancer, decrease depression, help with PMS, and even prevent you from getting sick.

Additionally, food can provide us with important vitamins, minerals, and phytonutrients. These include indole-3-carbinol and lignans, all of which help prevent certain cancers. Broccoli and brussels sprouts are examples of vegetables containing indole-3-carbinol. Lignans are found in flaxseeds, soybeans, and other seeds. Flavonoids, found in strawberries, spinach, and much more, are great as an anti-inflammatory.[1] So, eating the right foods can help us prevent cancer, battle inflammation, and provide ourselves with natural vitamins. They can do that and so much more!

When we talk about a "diet" we should be focusing more on a lifestyle. A lifestyle of eating whole foods instead of processed foods, eating food in a variety of colors, eating with the seasons, getting food at the farmers' markets, cooking at home, and minimizing empty calories. Examples of empty calories are: soda, slushies, cookies, candy, potato chips, and ice cream. Nutrient-dense foods include broccoli, salmon, spinach, nuts, and strawberries.

Have you ever noticed how you feel in the morning after binging on processed food the night before? Food has an effect on our mood. Eating too much sugar can lead to a crash shortly after, while drinking lots of caffeine might keep us from sleeping well. Our food choices can make or break our day.

Let's break down macronutrients. What are they?

Proteins, Carbohydrates, and Fats.

Protein

Protein in our diet is important for more than just body builders. Protein is important for making enzymes, antibodies which fight viruses, connective tissue and even neurotransmitters. Did you know that neurotransmitters like serotonin (made from tryptophan, an amino acid) help us feel calm and relaxed? Think of that happy feeling after a big turkey dinner.

It's recommended for adults to intake 0.36 grams of protein for every pound of body weight each day. For example: If you weigh 150 lbs. you would multiply 150 x .36 to calculate your daily protein need in grams. So, a 150 lb. adult would need about 54 grams of protein daily.

If you are over 60, it is recommended to have more protein per day to account for loss of muscle mass. For athletes, the recommended daily amount is doubled.

Healthier Protein Options

Choose This	Not That
Grass-Fed Beef	Grain-Fed Beef
Organic chicken	Regular factory-raised chicken
Wild salmon	Farmed salmon
Organic, free-range eggs	Egg substitutes and/or regular eggs

Carbohydrates

There are simple carbohydrates and complex carbohydrates. Certain types of dietary fiber are also considered carbohydrates. Carbohydrates vary in their effects on blood sugar levels. Their glycemic index is a way to quantify how they affect blood glucose levels after consumption. For example: baked potatoes, jelly beans, or white bread are rapidly digested and will cause a rapid increase in glucose levels (also increasing insulin levels in the blood). Oatmeal, apples, or broccoli are absorbed more slowly so the glucose levels rise more slowly while they are digested. It is important to consider picking foods with a lower glycemic index. This helps your body keep glucose levels steadier, and keeps you healthier!

Healthier Carbohydrate Options

Choose This	Instead of This
Sweet potato	Regular potato
Broccoli or Cauliflower rice	Rice
Black bean brownie	Regular brownie (with wheat flour)
Quinoa	Pasta

Fats

Fats are also important for our body. Besides helping with our basic bodily functions, fats are a key component of cell membranes and are precursors to biochemical mediators and hormone production. Dietary fats are classified based on the number of carbon-carbon bonds present in the fatty acids.

Saturated fats such as butter or coconut oil are solid at room temperature. Polyunsaturated fats include omega-3 and omega-6 fatty acids. Both are important for supporting proper, healthy brain and heart function. Keep in mind we need to have a proper ratio of omega-3 to omega-6.

Examples of oils high in omega-6 are sunflower oil, corn oil, and soybean oil. These should not be used for high-temperature cooking because they can form toxic lipid peroxides (basically, damaged lipid molecules). Unfortunately, however, soybean oil is frequently used in restaurants for frying foods. Omega-3 fatty acids have cardioprotective and anti-inflammatory effects. Having too much omega-6 fatty acids can throw off the balance in the body. We want a healthy ratio of omega-3 to omega-6 acids, or inflammation can occur. An example of healthy oil to cook with that is high in omega-3 fatty acids, is extra virgin olive oil. Avocado oil is another good oil to cook with (this also has monounsaturated fats which are good fats for the body).

We should completely avoid trans fatty acids that are artificial (like margarine). Trans fats have been linked to coronary artery disease (heart disease), an increase in total cholesterol, and lowering of HDL cholesterol (the good cholesterol).

Healthier Fat Options

Choose This	Not That
Olive oil	Canola Oil
Avocado Oil	Sunflower or Soy oil
Almond butter	Cream Cheese
Grass-fed butter (higher in gut-healthy butyric acid)	Butter (lower in omega-3 and vitamin K2)

By the Numbers

Now that we have a basic understanding of macronutrients, (Protein, Carbs, Fat) let's take a quick look at the caloric numbers, starting with the basics.

What's a calorie, anyway? In foods, a calorie is a unit of measurement. A calorie tells us the amount of energy required to raise 1 gram of water by 1-degree Celsius. So, we need to take in calories so our body can burn them so we can move and function. Different types of foods have different amounts of calories.

PROTEIN: 4 calories of energy per gram

<u>CARBS:</u> 4 calories of energy per gram

<u>FAT:</u> 9 calories of energy per gram

TYPES OF DIETS

L et's break down some of the more popular diets. Like we mentioned before, you want to focus on more of a lifestyle change than just a diet. Also, be careful with the word *diet*. More often than not, a *diet* leads to restriction and then binging. What's more important is to incorporate a lifestyle change that will lead to a better-quality life. Our goal is to help you eat your way to more energy and better health.

Mediterranean Diet

This popular diet is well studied for its protective effects from cardiovascular disease, boosting cognitive health (your brain's ability to think), and fighting against cancers. The many benefits of this diet most likely stem from the high amount of olive oil consumed with healthy omega-3. Let's break it down!

Vegetables: 4 or more servings each day

Fruits: 3 or more servings each day

Grains : 4 or more servings each day

Fats/Oils: Olive Oil - 4 Tablespoons or more each day

Nuts/Seeds: 3 or more servings each week

Beans/Legumes: 3 or more servings each week

Fish and Seafood: 2-3 servings each week

Herbs and Spices: use daily

Yogurt/Cheese/Egg Poultry: daily to weekly

Alcohol/Wine: Men — 1-2 glasses each day; Women — 1 glass each day

Here's an example of what a daily menu might look like if you were practicing the Mediterranean Diet:

Breakfast: steel-cut oats with blueberries and walnuts

Snack: banana or apple

Lunch: mixed greens, chickpeas, onions, carrots, olives, cucumbers, feta cheese, organic sprouted bread, salad dressing (olive oil & balsamic vinegar)

Dinner: salmon, brown rice, roasted broccoli in olive oil

Snack: almonds

Beverages: water, sparkling water, green tea, one glass of red wine

Atkins Diet

Atkins is a low-carbohydrate diet. Bacon for breakfast? Pork rinds for a snack? It's easy to see why this diet garnered a lot of popularity when it was introduced by cardiologist Robert Atkins, MD. The Atkins Diet emphasizes animal foods, eggs, cheese, and low-carbohydrate vegetables. It does not restrict caloric intake. Two things to consider with the Atkins Diet are: The low carb intake can greatly help with quicker weight loss; however, the long-term safety is still questionable with this diet lifestyle. This means, for a short term, this might not damage our heart or kidneys, but in the long term it might do harm.

Here's an example of what a daily menu might look like eating the Atkins Diet:

Breakfast: bacon and eggs

Snack: carrots or celery with ranch salad dressing

Lunch: flank steak, broccoli cooked in olive oil

Snack: low carb snack bar

Dinner: hamburger (no bun), pepperjack cheese, avocado, lettuce, sliced tomato

Beverages: water, tea, no-calorie drinks

Paleo Diet

Eating like a caveman? That's the gist of the Paleo Diet. Early humans were primarily hunters and gatherers. They didn't regularly harvest grains and they weren't baking bread. If our paleolithic ancestors didn't eat it, we shouldn't either if we're following this diet. In people on the Paleo Diet, studies have shown improvement in weight loss, blood pressure, and triglycerides.[2] This diet places an emphasis on foods that can be hunted (fish and meat) or gathered (tree nuts, eggs, vegetables, fruits, berries). Raw honey, coconut sugar, olive oil, ghee, and coconut oil are all acceptable. Dairy, grains, sugar, legumes, rice, white potatoes, and processed oils are all strictly avoided.

The daily menu while practicing the Paleo Diet might include:

<u>Breakfast</u>: spinach omelet cooked in coconut oil, raspberries

<u>Snack</u>: apple and almond butter

<u>Lunch</u>: chicken salad, avocado, onions, fresh blueberries

<u>Dinner</u>: steak, cauliflower rice with coconut amines, roasted sweet potato

<u>Snack</u>: dates with walnuts

<u>Beverages</u>: water, herbal tea, coffee

Vegetarian Diet

Let's make one key distinction: Vegan vs. Vegetarian. What's the difference?

<u>Vegan</u>: Consumes no animal products. Period.

<u>Vegetarian</u>: Does not eat animals, but may eat products that come from animals (eggs, dairy, honey)

The Vegetarian Diet is fairly self-explanatory. Load up on plenty of fruits, vegetables, legumes, and healthy grains, but do keep in mind, while vegetarians have a lower incidence of cardiovascular disease, hypertension, kidney stones, and diabetes (compared to most omnivores), they may be low in micronutrients. If you follow a Vegetarian Diet, some supplementation may be necessary to ensure you're getting sufficient amounts of vitamin B12, iron, vitamin D, zinc, iodine, riboflavin, calcium, and selenium.[3]

Along with a bevy of vegetables, here are some popular food choices for the Vegetarian Diet:

- quinoa and pumpkin seeds
- all-natural nut butter on whole-grain bread
- rice and beans
- soybeans with soba noodles
- Ezekiel bread with almond butter
- brown rice with mushrooms and herbs

Low-FODMAPs Diet

"FODMAPs" is an acronym for Fermentable Oligosaccharides, Disaccharides, Monosaccharides, And Polyols. I know what you may be thinking. In plain English, please.

At its most basic, the Low FODMAP[4] Diet cuts out certain carbohydrates that can cause or trigger irritable bowel syndrome (IBS). This diet is low in FODMAPs which include fructose, lactose, sorbitol, fructans (fructooligosaccharides, inulin), and galactans (also called galactooligosaccharides; e.g., raffinose). It's been shown to help, and often improve the symptoms, of patients with irritable bowel syndrome, bloating, or abdominal pain., often improving their symptoms.

Here's an example of eating the Low-FODMAP diet:
   Breakfast: steel-cut oats, almond milk, strawberries
   Snack: pumpkin seeds and cucumber slices
   Lunch: salmon, quinoa, spinach, olive oil
   Dinner: grilled chicken with spaghetti squash and tomato sauce
   Snack: 1-piece dairy-free >70% dark chocolate

AIP Diet

The autoimmune protocol diet (AIP) is a strict diet used to help decrease inflammation in the body and improve gut health. You are allowed to eat vegetables (except for nightshades), fruits, protein, and healthy fats. However, on the AIP diet, you strictly avoid grains, dairy, soy, nuts, seeds, legumes, nightshades, eggs, additives, and artificial sugars.

That's quite a list! But on the bright side, studies have shown the AIP Diet improves symptoms in patients suffering from irritable bowel syndrome (IBS)[5] and decreases inflammatory markers.[6]

An example of eating the AIP Diet:

Breakfast: turkey sausage with blueberries

Snack: apples and cucumber slices

Lunch: salmon salad with olive oil dressing

Dinner: Chicken Marsala (use tapioca starch)

Snack: bone broth with chicken, carrots, celery, and onions

Ketogenic Diet

Often called Keto, the Ketogenic Diet was originally used to help patients with seizure disorders. Now, the Keto Diet is very popular for effective weight loss. Like the Atkins, the Keto is higher in fats and protein, allows low amounts of carbs, but there are other benefits to this diet. The Ketogenic Diet promotes a non-atherogenic lipid profile, lowers blood pressure, and improves glucose and insulin levels.[7] What this means is, the cholesterol is going to be less likely to form plaques, which lead to heart disease and heart attacks. This diet also has antineoplastic (anti-cancer) benefits. It's been shown not to alter renal or liver function or produce metabolic acidosis, meaning those on this diet will have lab work still in a normal range. Ketosis has possible neurological benefits in the central nervous system, including decreasing inflammation, while slowing osteoporosis. If that's not enough, the Keto Diet may even increase performance in aerobic sports, like swimming, running, and Zumba.

Here's an example of a daily menu eating the Ketogenic Diet:

Breakfast: eggs cooked in coconut oil with bacon

Snack: grass-fed beef stick

Lunch: grilled salmon on romaine lettuce with avocado oil ranch dressing

Dinner: grass-fed steak with a side of broccoli cooked in butter

Snack: hardboiled egg

Beverages: water, tea, butter coffee

Whole 30 Diet

The Whole-30 Diet is an elimination-style eating plan that eliminates common trigger foods. Soy, dairy, grains, alcohol, legumes, and added sugars are strictly removed from the diet. After 30 days, when the body is at a baseline, these foods are slowly introduced back into the diet one at a time. This allows you to take note of any particular foods that cause allergic or inflammatory responses of which you were not previously aware. By eliminating foods for 30 days, you can now note any negative effects those trigger foods have on your body.

Here's an example of what a menu looks like on the Whole-30 Diet:

<u>Breakfast</u>: smoked salmon and poached eggs

<u>Snack</u>: mixed nuts and salami

<u>Lunch</u>: taco lettuce wraps with plantain chips and salsa

<u>Dinner</u>: zucchini noodles with avocado pesto and shrimp

<u>Snack</u>: dates and walnuts (or a fruit and nut bar such as Larabar™)

<u>Beverages</u>: purified water

Intermittent & Modified Fasting

Fasting is typically seen as a hypo-caloric diet. Hypo-caloric is just a fancy way of saying there's a reduction of daily food or calories. Dietary restriction means purposely not eating at certain times of the day or evening. That may explain why there are different strategies of when to eat and when to fast. How long should the fasting window be?

In short, fasting means not eating any food. Consuming water, black coffee, and tea may be allowed, so long as they do not contain calories. But keep in mind, some religious fasting does not allow consumption of anything during the fasting window.

Traditional Fasting has been part of religious ceremonies for thousands of years. Traditional fasting restricts eating between certain periods of the day. In these religious ceremonies, the number of calories is typically reduced because the number of hours to consume the meals is reduced.

Clinical Fasting is fasting typically done under medical supervision with a low daily caloric intake (200–900 kcal nutritional intake/day) for periods of 7 to 21 days. Done under clinical supervision, this fast has been shown to help with medical issues such as depression and rheumatoid arthritis.[8]

Intermittent Fasting can be thought of as time-restricted eating. In a 24-hour period, there is a small window of time for eating and a larger window of time for fasting. The benefits and results of intermittent fasting may vary depending on the number and timing of meals. Additionally, portioning the entire intake into two meals without changing the total energy consumption may have beneficial effects on the inflammatory markers of metabolic syndrome.[9] An example would be waiting to eat until noon.

Intermittent fasting and reducing total timing of food consumption (time-restricted eating) appears to have some of the same results as traditional fasting, such as reducing oxidative stress and decreasing pro-inflammatory cytokines (the bad inflammation)[10].

There are lots of benefits to an intermittent fast. It could be as simple as having an earlier dinner and skipping breakfast the next day. Time-restricted and intermittent fasting are commonly practiced by using an "eating window." In a 24-hour day, you fast for 16 consecutive hours and then eat during the next 8 hours. That would be a 16:8 window, 16 off, 8 on. Another common practice is an 18:6 window. 18 hours fasting, 6 hours eating. More extreme examples are 20:4 or even 22:2. But whatever you choose, it's recommended to have at least 12 hours of fasting overnight to allow the gut to rest and for autophagy (recycling or removing old cell material), to take place. The process of autophagy is crucial for a healthy bod

Intermittent fasting is easier than you think.

Here's an example of a 16:8 fast. Your eating window is noon-8pm:

Breakfast: skip. Drink water, organic tea, organic black coffee

Lunch: eat something sensible (such as an omelet, smoothie, or salmon salad) starting at 12 pm

Snack: whatever you'd like, as needed (such as almonds or a grass-fed beef stick)

Dinner: something sensible, but nothing after 8pm

WHICH DIET IS RIGHT FOR ME?

If you are looking to try one of these diets, contact your physician and a dietician before you make any major lifestyle changes. Your local library is also a great resource. Internet searches for more information about these specific diets may be helpful. There are countless books and reputable magazines that can offer more detailed information on each of these diets. You can also find a host of tasty menu ideas, meal plans, and delicious recipes online and in print.

Do keep this in mind though, whichever diet you try, you will want to stick with it for at least one month to receive the benefits. Remember, make it a lifestyle. This isn't a fad. It's a choice for you and your family to live healthier and more active lives.

The Usual Suspects

After you eat out, do you sometimes feel like junk? Do you find yourself wanting to take a power nap after that drive-thru lunch? Ask yourself, what are you putting into your body? If it's processed food, toxins, and refined sugars, there's a reason your body feels that oncoming crash. Garbage in. Garbage out.

So, what should you avoid? What should go into your shopping cart and what should stay on the shelf? Let's answer these questions.

We've covered some foods that can benefit our health and others that are toxic to our bodies. But what exactly makes some foods so bad for us? After all, a calorie is just a calorie.

Unfortunately, our body doesn't process all calories the same. When our body is faced with chemicals it doesn't need, it will put precious energy into detoxing and purging instead of focusing on keeping the body healthy. This can mean decreased energy, decreased immune function, and increased stress on the body. Foods we should avoid can also cause us to pack on pounds and become overweight. Not good!

Let's look at some of the usual suspects in greater detail. If you see these on the label, don't even think about it. Put it back on the shelf.

Artificial Dyes

Ever wondered why your children acted out after a Halloween party? Why were they acting crazy at that birthday party? Why was their sleep off? Well, food dyes could be to blame.

Artificial food dyes are chemicals not found in natural food sources. We are naturally attracted to bright colors. We reach for brightly colored packages over plain colored ones. The same goes for what we put in our mouth. However, when it comes to food dyes, it comes at a price.

So which dyes have been shown to cause negative outcomes?

Meet public enemy number one: **Yellow No. 5**

This bad boy is loaded into candy, breakfast cereals, sodas, and much more. It gives a yellow color but can also be used in green items. Studies show this food dye (also called tartrazine), when combined with sodium benzoate (a common food preservative), can cause irritability, restlessness, and sleep disturbances in children.[11] Is your child eating this each morning in their breakfast cereal? What about that popsicle, or that fruit-flavored drink? Better read that label again. It might be time to swap out those candy-colored fruit loops so your child can have a better day at school.

Are you seeing red? Look out for this suspect: **Red dye 40**.

Red dye 40 is found in a variety of foods from Doritos™, and M&Ms™, to salad dressing. This additive is proven to increase hyperactivity in children.[12]

Ask any teacher after a classroom birthday party with red icing cupcakes; it's something worse than just a sugar high. And it's only getting worse. The consumption of artificial food coloring has quadrupled in the past 50 years.[13] These chemicals also affect the brain and should be avoided if possible. In the words of the Greek philosopher, Paracelsus, "The dose makes the poison."

So, what should we do? First, check the label on the products you consume. Avoid additives altogether if you can. Look for natural colorings such as spirulina, beetroot, and turmeric. And consider this last nugget when making your food choices: When children with ADHD (attention-deficit/hyperactivity disorder) were put on an elimination diet, taking out preservatives and artificial colorings, they showed improvement in ADHD symptoms.

Artificial Flavorings & Additives

It might not be your fault that you want to eat McDonald's all the time. And there's a good reason why, once you pop that can of chips, you can't stop shoving them into your face. These foods are chemically engineered to trigger our brains. Like an addictive drug, they make us crave more, even though they are not good for our bodies. The hidden culprit is food additives. They've been shown to increase

ADHD symptoms in children. Even worse, some studies are suggesting food additives may be part of the cause of ADHD[14].

So, what is a food additive? In short, it's something added to your food to enhance its taste, flavor, or appearance. Some examples are nitrites, nitrates, potassium bromate, BHT, propylparaben, and diacetyl, but one of the most dangerous forms of food additives is hiding in plain sight.

Sugar. Did you know sugar activates the same pleasure areas of your brain as cocaine? It's true. Sugar is highly pleasurable and equally addictive, and that might be part of the reason why it's everywhere. It's in your coffee, your ketchup, your soup, your bread, but it's even worse than that. Sugar is called a lot of things when added to foods. It hides under other aliases like corn syrup, high fructose corn syrup, malt sugar, turbinado sugar, glucose, cane syrup, fructose, mannose, sugar beet, and more.

So why is sugar so bad?

First, sugar is very inflammatory. Americans consume 16.1% of their total calories from added sugars, and that problem is only getting worse.[15] Because sugar is addictive and we crave it, we have a hard time cutting sugar out. And our craving for sugar leads us to binge eat high-sugar foods[16].

On the tongue, sugar is highly palatable. It's an instant reward, both in taste and its nutritive input but there's danger involved. Consuming excessive sugar triggers neuroadaptations in the reward system that decouples eating behavior from caloric needs. This means sugar targets the part of the brain that causes pleasure, the part that drugs affect. In plain English, you eat way more of it than you need (e.g., that empty pint of Ben & Jerry's™ ice cream).

The science behind overeating and sugar is alarming. There is a clear link between regularly eating high-sugar foods and compulsive overeating. Excessive sugar intake is, in turn, associated with adverse health conditions, including obesity, high blood pressure, diabetes, bad cholesterol, and heart disease.[17]

In a study of rats eating sugar, researchers concluded sugar was more addictive than cocaine.[18] The rats' brains were more rewarded when regularly given sugar than when regularly given cocaine. The rats chose the sweet, sugar-sweetened substance over highly addictive cocaine[19]. In summary, when regularly eaten, sweets are very addictive.

Most studies are concerned with added sugar. Additives like sucrose and fructose are widely studied. These additives were not in our ancestors' diets, but they are found in most processed foods. The more sugars and additives we eat, the more we crave. We are constantly stuck in that hamster wheel, running after that next sugar high. When we consider the evidence linking high sugar consumption to obesity, metabolic syndrome, and the development of diabetes, this is a catastrophic feedback loop.

But it gets worse. Say hello to **high fructose corn syrup (HFCS).**

If sugar is a wave, high fructose corn syrup is a tsunami. This additive crash your health and that of your children. It's cheap. It's manufactured. It's in everything.

HFCS is linked to a higher rate of obesity and an increased risk of colorectal cancer[20]. The other concern is high fructose corn syrup's involvement in the development of nonalcoholic fatty liver disease (NASH)[21]. Beverages containing high fructose corn syrup, such as soda, have been linked to weight gain and increased risk of obesity, simply by drinking soda for just 6 months[22]. One study showed the visceral fat, the "spare tire" of fat around your waist, was the area affected the most. This type of fat is the most harmful type of body fat and is linked to health issues such as heart disease and diabetes. Consuming food or drinks with HFCS can also increase inflammation in the body and increase the risk for gout, a painful joint disease.[23] Fructose has also been noted to increase food-seeking and increased fat production and fat storage.[24] Another concern is the link between high fructose corn syrup and fatty liver disease.

Nonalcoholic liver disease (liver disease not caused by drinking alcohol) can lead to liver cirrhosis. Yes, liver failure. High fructose corn syrup is bad news. Do not take it lightly. It's best to stay away from this addictive food additive.

PROCESSED FOODS & HIGH GLYCEMIC INDEX

Here's the problem with quick, cheap, processed foods. They're packed with additives, sugars, and preservatives, and after we eat them, they often leave us hungry again within an hour. Foods with a high glycemic index will raise your blood sugar quickly (which also raises your insulin) and lead to a crash in energy levels. If you pick a low glycemic index food (think foods with more fat and fiber), you will feel fuller longer. You'll feel steadier and won't experience that crash.

Not only does eating processed foods with a high glycemic index make you feel bad, but it can also cause drastic fluctuations in your blood glucose levels. This can eventually lead to the development of diabetes. This is why it's essential to choose foods with a lower glycemic index. These food choices have more fiber in them. When offered a choice, go for fresh foods over dried foods. Fresh fruits, for example, contain more fiber and are usually a lower glycemic index than dried foods. Think of eating a handful of grapes versus a handful of raisins. I'm sure you've noticed, when you're hungry you eat fewer grapes to feel full than if you're snacking on raisins. The same goes for juices. How many oranges do you eat to feel satisfied versus how many it takes to make a glass of orange juice?

Low Glycemic Index Foods (Green= Go)

Broccoli, Celery, Peas

Apple, Pear, Grapes

Carrots, Black beans

Medium Glycemic Index Foods (Yellow = Caution)

Corn, Banana

Sweet potato, White rice

Raisins, Table sugar

High Glycemic Index Foods ("Red" = Stop)

White bread, Potatoes

French fries, Doughnuts

Jelly beans, Dates

Artificial Sweeteners

We know sugar is bad for us, so maybe grabbing a diet soda would seem like the next best option. Not so fast!

Artificial sweeteners are also bad news. Most are highly processed. Stay away from sucralose, aspartame, and Splenda. Not only are they riddled with chemicals, but they also might make you fat! Yes, you read that right.

Researchers in one study looked at the link between artificial sweeteners and obesity. It appears artificial sweeteners change your gut microbiome, leading to problems with glucose, and consuming them will increase overall caloric intake.[25] It seems counterintuitive, but trying to save calories by consuming fake sugar can actually cause more damage.

Caffeine & Alcohol

Like most things in life, use these in moderation, and in this case, also use caution. These drugs have different effects on the body. Caffeine is a stimulant, while alcohol is a depressant. Caffeine is an addictive food and can increase anxiety in some users. Obviously, if it's consumed later in the day it can interfere with sleep. If you are going to have your coffee in the morning, consider swapping it out for something healthier. Give green tea a try, but try to limit yourself to just one cup.

Alcohol has its own side effects to consider. Excessive alcohol intake contributes to a number of health concerns: hepatitis, cirrhosis, cardiomyopathy, depression, dementia, and nutritional deficiencies. However, it is widely believed that moderate alcohol consumption (1 drink per day for women, 2 drinks per day for men) isn't harmful for most people. In fact, some studies show a small drink may reduce the risk of developing cardiovascular disease. Otherwise known as "The French Paradox" it is thought one glass of wine which has antioxidants might be helpful.[26] Never the less, the purported cardioprotective effect of alcohol is based primarily on observational studies and is still open to debate. The message is simple: When it comes to consuming addictive substances like caffeine and alcohol, caution must be observed.

Pesticides & Herbicides

This one is simple. If an insect doesn't want to eat the vegetation because it's been sprayed with a poison, you probably don't want to ingest it either. The serious and grave health risks of pesticides and herbicides have been widely described. You've probably even seen a commercial or two about cancer lawsuits involving weed killers. Again, you don't want to be ingesting added chemicals. Our concern is how can we avoid these poisons on our food? What can you do to avoid pesticides while grocery shopping?

For starters, go to the Environmental Working Group, or EWG.org website and download the shopping list for fruits and vegetables. They've trademarked them as the *Clean 15* and the *Dirty 12*. Write them down (they change seasonally) and pick up the clean ones when you go grocery shopping. Easy fix. If the recommended foods are not available where you shop, there are still steps you can take to mitigate exposure to pesticides.

Obviously, buying organic helps. Organic producers have stricter guidelines to follow in the production of their foods, however, being certified organic does not mean the food is chemical and pesticide-free at harvest. When you get your produce home, make sure you wash it off. A vinegar soak is ideal. Enough said.

High Dietary Salt Intake

Sodium by itself can be deadly. Chloride on its own is lethal. When you chemically combine them, you get sodium chloride, table salt, an essential mineral in a healthy diet. Such is the magic of chemistry. A high intake of salt is associated with an increased risk of obesity and hypertension. Those factors can lead to an increased risk of stroke and heart attack.[27]

The World Health Organization (WHO) recommends salt consumption levels of less than 5 grams each day, but it has been estimated that the current intake of salt in most countries of the world is 9-12 grams daily.

Why is this a problem?

It's estimated 50-60% of people with hypertension are salt-sensitized. There is research suggesting the elderly and overweight populations gain the most benefit from decreasing their salt intake. Reduce your salt and you can reduce the risk for cardiovascular disease.[28] One diet, the Dietary Approaches to Stop Hypertension (DASH), has been helpful for people at risk of cardiovascular disease. The DASH diet recommends foods lower in sodium and foods rich in potassium, magnesium, and calcium. These nutrients also aid in lowering blood pressure. On this diet, you consume vegetables, fruits, whole grains, fish, poultry, and nuts. And in moderation, you can add meats, red wine, and even some sweets.

Salt is definitely needed in our diet and is a great way to add flavor to vegetables, but it's the hidden sodium, the salt added to processed foods, that can be harmful to our long-term health. If you're cooking your own food, season lightly. If you're eating processed food, read the labels carefully. How many grams of salt are hiding in there?

Helpful Hint:

A pinch of salt contains about 400 mg of sodium!

Soybean & Canola Oils

If you look at a bottle of vegetable oil, it will claim it's great for making salad dressing, which might lead you to believe it's a healthy ingredient. Guess what? These oils aren't good for you. In fact, soybean oil has been linked to obesity and diabetes.

A recent study of mice found that feeding them soybean oil showed profound effects on the hypothalamus, the part of the brain that regulates metabolism and hunger among many other functions.[29] The soybean-fed mice developed health issues including obesity, diabetes, insulin resistance, and fatty liver disease. Scientists have also linked soybean oil to neurological conditions like autism, depression, anxiety, and even Alzheimer's disease. Levels of oxytocin went down in mice that were fed soybean oil. Oxytocin is produced in the hypothalamus and is known as the love hormone.

So think about it, you eat a bunch of fries cooked in rancid GMO (genetically modified organism) soybean oil from the fast food place, your hypothalamus goes haywire, your feel-good oxytocin hormone goes down, you get sad, and to deal with that feeling of woe, you go stuff more fries in your mouth. Then what? You start feeling like junk. You get sluggish and gain a bunch of weight, but you're sitting there depressed, ordering more fried food to feel better.

Now you're depressed, and obese, and have insulin resistance and fatty liver disease. No wonder we're popping Zoloft like breath mints. (Zoloft is an antidepressant classified as a Selective Serotonin Reuptake Inhibitor (SSRI.) Do yourself (and your liver) a favor, pass on foods cooked in soybean oil.

What about canola oil?

Like other vegetable oils, canola oil is highly processed. It goes through a process of refining to make it an oil that involves chemicals to bleach the rapeseed first, and chemicals for degumming. The solvent manufacturers typically use hexane. In the final steps of the refinement process, the oil is deodorized, which involves even more chemicals.

Oils that are cold-pressed are better, but these are harder to find and more expensive. Canola and soybean oil are cheap to make. That's why you see them in many cheap, convenient food products. Cold-pressed oils are made by the physical pressing of the products instead of using heat and chemicals. A few examples of cold-pressed oils include: Avocado oil and olive oil. Let's make this simple. Avoid these highly processed, chemical-filled foods. Just think of the inflammation they'll cause in your body.

STRATEGIES FOR GROCERY SHOPPING

L et's keep this simple, too. Consider these two principles when you shop at the grocery store:

Buy food.

Don't buy products.

To accomplish this, stay on the perimeter of the grocery store. This is where you'll find the healthier foods, produce, fruits, meats, and fish. It's the inner aisles where you'll get into trouble. The inside aisles of most grocery stores are filled with a maze of processed food, including chips, cereals, canned goods loaded with salt, or frozen meals full of preservatives. Stay out of the middle. Be an outsider!

Most grocery stores now have organic options next to the regular items. Choose organic when you can. There will be fewer pesticides and unnecessary ingredients. If you *have* to buy processed foods, read the labels. Avoid food dyes, artificial flavors, bad oils, and hidden sugars. Most food products that come in a package will be loaded with junk.

Beware of salad dressings. When you read the label, you'll find that many of them contain additives. Keep an eye out for high fructose corn syrup, food dyes, bad oils, and sodium. If you're shopping with your family, ask them to help out. Have them read the labels with you; for kids, make it a game. Look for hidden oils, hidden artificial food coloring, or hidden sugar. Now that you're looking for them, you will be amazed at how many of those products are hiding in foods.

Limit buying snacks like potato chips, soda pop, sweets, and fruit snacks. They're packed full of junk. If it's in the house, you or someone in your family will be tempted to eat it. Instead, save those items for special occasions.

Focus on veggies and fresh fruit and your body will thank you. Sometimes frozen vegetables are a great option. Since they are picked fresh and then quickly frozen, they can still have great flavor even if they are out of season. Remember, the first time you shop for healthy foods may take you longer since you're reading the labels. The more you do it, the easier it will become.

Another great way to shop for produce is to utilize your local farmers' market. By shopping for farm-to-table food, you are supporting your local economy. You can find all the vegetables you need there, fresh and in season. Plus, most markets carry other local items like berries, eggs, meat, and honey. Check to see where and when your farmers' market occurs and make it a habit to visit.

Let's recap. Use these strategies at the grocery store to make stronger food choices:

- Stay on the perimeter
- Read the labels.
- Load up on veggies
- Buy food, not products

Food as Medicine

CP came to me after being diagnosed with colon cancer. He was frustrated with his energy levels and wanted to optimize his health while going through cancer treatments. Unfortunately, his cancer doctors were not giving him sound advice on nutrition. When he came to me, he was following their instructions and still eating canned and processed foods. I spoke with him about how nutrition is key for health and to think of food as medicine. And it's true, what we put into our bodies will either heal disease or create disease. Everything we put in our mouths is going to help fight cancer or promote cancer. Each bite will reduce inflammation or produce inflammation.

After our talk, CP changed his diet. He eliminated the highly processed foods. He invested in a juicer. Most importantly, he paid more attention to how the foods he ate made him feel. To round things off, we helped CP by also adding supplements to support his digestion. He worked hard changing his diet and increasing anti-inflammatory foods. And the work paid off. By making better food choices, CP felt better and had more energy.

For his follow up appointment, I was floored when he walked in the door. He looked amazing and his cancer was stable. What a difference our fuel makes! By focusing on simple nutritional habits CP was feeling so much better. Good, healthy food is the glue that holds a healthy body together.

Let's Get Cooking

If cooking was easy, everybody would save money and do it. The truth is, it can take a lot of work to cook your own meals. With our busy schedules, home cooking can be over-whelming, but it can also be rewarding and a lot of fun.

To make healthy meals at home, you only need a stovetop, oven, pans, and a few other basic cooking utensils and goods. Olive oil is a great fat. You can use it to sauté, roast, and bake. Olive oil is also packed with heart-healthy omega-3 fatty acids.

Crockpots are a great tool for cooking at home, for example, when making nutrient-dense chili at home. Beans are a great source of protein and fiber. Tomatoes are packed with phytonutrients such as lycopene. Add in grass-fed meat for protein and onions for vitamin c and folate. Toss all your ingredients into the pot in the morning and it's done for dinner! Another great use for the crockpot is easy shredded chicken. Place the chicken breast in the crockpot in the morning, and get shredded chicken when you get home from work. It's great on salads, in casseroles, and more. Chicken thighs (contain more fat) cook perfectly also.

Instapots are also great kitchen tools for the reluctant chef. Cooking vegetables in the Instapot is one of the best ways to cook vegetables since more nutrients are retained. Instapots can also steam rice, cook quinoa, meat, chicken, and much more. You can even make homemade soup stocks and bone broths in the Instapot.

In summation, don't be afraid to get in the kitchen and give home cooking a try. It's easier than you think. Heat up your veggies until they are tender and season them lightly. Toss some greens with a few of your favorite chopped vegetables and herbs and drizzle with some olive oil and dash of vinegar. That's all there is to it. You're on your way.

RECIPE IDEAS

Here are a few recipes to get you started. For more ideas and international flavors, browse the internet, visit a book store, or peruse your local library. There are millions of recipes at your fingertips.

Salad Dressing

½ cup extra virgin olive oil

¼ cup apple cider vinegar

½ cup local honey

1 tsp dried basil

¼ tsp sea salt

Mix together and serve on a salad.

GF/DF Banana Bread

(makes two loaves)

2 cups gluten-free flour blend (or almond flour + 1/2 tsp xanthan gum)

1 tsp baking soda

1/2 tsp salt

6 overripe bananas, mashed

2 eggs

1 1/2 cups organic sugar

1/2 cup organic maple syrup

1/2 cup melted coconut oil

1/2 cup dairy free chocolate chips

(I added a touch of ground flaxseed and oatmeal to boost my milk production because I am breastfeeding, but these are healthy for everyone!)

Mash the bananas first, add the "wet" ingredients, then add the dry ingredients. Mix and pour batter into two loaf pans. Bake at 350 degrees for 45 - 60 minutes (until a toothpick comes out clean)

Baking with small kids means making recipes simple and in one bowl! It still turns out yummy!

Homemade Gummies

1 cup 100% organic fruit juice

2-3 tbsp honey

6 tbsp gelatin

Add fruit juice, honey, and gelatin in a pan on the stove and heat until warm and all the gelatin is dissolved.

Use medicine droppers to transfer to molds, or pour into molds.

Place in the fridge until solid.

Push out of the molds and refrigerate what you don't use

Tips: Add the gelatin slowly while mixing so it won't clump together. For your beverage, pick a fruit juice with no added sugar.

Cucumber Cilantro Salad

2 cucumbers peeled and sliced

1 chopped onion

Fresh cilantro (as you prefer)

Lime juice (from one lime)

2 tsp apple cider vinegar

4 tsp extra virgin olive oil

1/2 tsp garlic powder and a touch of Celtic salt

Mix together and it's ready to serve.

So refreshing for the summer and you can even put it in a glass mason jar and pack it for lunch.

"Iron Cookies" (Molasses cookies which are high in iron)

1/2 cup organic brown sugar

1/2 cup coconut oil (melted)

2 free-range, organic eggs

1/4 cup blackstrap molasses

1 tsp ginger

1 tsp cinnamon

1 tsp non-aluminum baking soda

1 1/2 cup GF flour blend

You can plop these onto a baking sheet by the tablespoonful and sprinkle some sugar on top, or you can place in the refrigerator for an hour.

Take them out, roll into balls, roll each in sugar and flatten on baking sheet.

Bake at 350 degrees for 10 minutes

Chickpea Chocolate Chip Cookie Dough

1 can chickpeas (drained and rinsed well)

1 tsp vanilla extract

1/3 cup nut butter (almond, cashew, or peanut butter)

¼ cup brown sugar (may substitute with honey, maple syrup or coconut sugar)

2 tsp ground flaxseed or oatmeal

(optional 1-3 Tbsp almond milk if you need a smoother consistency)

Add all the ingredients (except for the chocolate chips) to a food processor and blend until smooth consistency. Then mix in the chocolate chips. (Enjoy Life™ mini chips are my favorite!)

Store in the fridge and share (or don't share) with the family.

Black Bean Brownies

2 cans black beans, rinsed well

¼ cup oatmeal

½ cup natural sugar (I used a mix of maple syrup and honey)

2 eggs

½ cup raw cacao powder

¼ cup coconut oil, melted

1 tsp nonaluminum baking powder

Blend all ingredients in a food processor until smooth.

Grease with coconut oil or line an 8" x 8" baking pan with parchment paper

Bake at 350 degrees for 30 – 35 minutes.

Top with chocolate chips.

Share with friends and don't tell them the secret ingredient.

Golden Milk

2 cups unsweetened coconut milk

2 tsp raw honey

1/2 tsp cinnamon

1 tsp turmeric

Stir while bringing to a low boil on the stove.

Let cool to drinking temperature and enjoy.

Play around with the recipe and make it your own.

Maple syrup can be used instead of honey.

Almond milk can be used instead of coconut milk.

Egg Roll in a Bowl

6-8 cups shredded cabbage

1/2 - 1 lb ground sausage

1 onion, diced

1 cup carrot, shredded

Optional ingredients:

1/4 cup sprouts

1/2 cup green peas

1 egg, scrambled

Top with coconut amines or GF soy sauce

Cook sausage in a pan and set aside.

Scramble egg and set aside.

Sautee vegetables, stirring frequently, until cooked

Mix all ingredients together and serve with gluten-free soy sauce or coconut amines

Peanut Butter Pie

8 oz dairy-free cream cheese (the cleanest you can find)

1/2 tub of dairy-free whipped cream

1/2 cup peanut butter

1/4 cup coconut sugar

1/4 cup maple syrup

Place all ingredients in a bowl and mix well.

Place in a serving bowl and top with organic chocolate syrup and dairy-free chocolate chips.

You can use graham crackers to dip, or pour mix in a gluten-free graham cracker crust.

If you pour in a premade gluten free graham cracker crust, refrigerate for 4 hours before serving!

Chicken Paprikash

2 lbs organic chicken

1 onion

6 tbsp butter, ghee or coconut oil

1 carton (32 oz.) organic chicken stock or bone broth (bone broth can be made at home!)

8 oz. dairy-free sour cream (or regular sour cream)

4 - 6 tbsp paprika

Cut chicken breast into bite-size pieces, set aside

Place 4 tbsp butter or ghee into an oven-safe pan and sauté onions until soft.

Add 2 tbsp more of butter or ghee and add chicken. Cook on both sides until brown

Add chicken stock, sour cream, and paprika. Mix well.

Cook at 350 degrees for 45 minutes.

Serve with gluten-free pasta

One Last Reminder on Diet...

Say yes!	No way!
Whole, unprocessed foods	Refined sugars, refined carbs
Grass-fed beef	Trans fat, fast food
Organic, free-range eggs and chicken	Factory eggs and chicken
Organic fruits and vegetables	Canned fruits and veggies with added sugar and salt
Herbs and spices to enhance flavors	Food additives and salt
Sparkling water and tea	Excessive caffeine and alcohol

Final Thoughts

I know this seems like a lot of information, but even the smallest of actions can have an incredible impact on your health. Start small, but be consistent. Make one positive change each day for your health. Try to introduce one healthy food a month and cut out one unhealthy food a month. Try a new recipe each week and eat out one less time a week.

Pause before you buy something from the grocery store. Start reading the labels while you shop for groceries. Think twice before you order food when eating out. If you are eating out, look at the nutritional information and make an informed choice. When in doubt, just pick a protein and a steamed vegetable as a side. If you are going to order a salad, ask for olive oil and vinegar (or bring your own dressing with you). Swap out soda for an unsweetened tea. Drink plenty of clean, filtered water daily.

Children can be challenging, but if they see you eating healthy, they will follow your example. Continue to give them new fruits and vegetables; they might even learn to like foods they usually wouldn't eat before. Roasting, steaming, and sautéing are all different ways to cook your vegetables. Mix it up. Healthy food doesn't have to be boring!

And remember, food is medicine. What you put in your mouth is either creating inflammation or protecting your body against it. Consider what fuel you're putting in your tank.

SLEEP

The following is an example of work-related sleep deprivation.

BB was a workaholic. He spent most of his day focusing on the different aspects of his job and paying little attention to himself. The one thing which became obvious was how regularly BB was exhausted. It got to the point where BB started snapping at co-workers and he became someone that others in his office wanted to avoid. When I saw BB for exhaustion, he was convinced that something was physically wrong with him. He wondered if he had cancer or was anemic. He believed there had to be a medical explanation.

When I began questioning his lifestyle, he noted that, on average, he worked 12-14-hour days in the office and would often go home and continue working on his computer or watch TV until he fell asleep. He also noted he did not exercise and drank caffeine until 8 pm so he could get a little more work in before bedtime, which was usually around 1 am. Many nights he would have 2 bourbon on the rocks nightcaps, which he felt helped him sleep. On average, BB slept about 4-5 hours a night. His philosophy was, "I can sleep when I am dead."

This, unfortunately, is a much more common scenario than we would like to believe. We spend approximately a third of our lives asleep.[30] That's great news if you're waking up refreshed after a deep and soothing rest. Unfortunately, many of us are not practicing good sleep habits. As a result, we may suffer from chronic fatigue, health issues, and low performance in our daily lives. This is an all-too-common problem. Approximately 30% of adults have one or more symptoms of insomnia,[31] while 20-30% of infants, toddlers, and preschoolers experience frequent nighttime awakenings or bedtime problems.[32]

The National Sleep Foundation 2014 Sleep Health Index ™ found that 45% of American adults reported they had poor or insufficient sleep affecting their daily activities at least once in the past seven days.[33] Another study by the University of Pennsylvania Perelman School of Medicine found that 25% of Americans experience acute insomnia each year, but 75% will recover without developing chronic insomnia.[34] Even though the percent recovery from insomnia sounds promising, a 2007 study found that self-reported complaints of insomnia were associated with an increased risk of coronary artery disease, heart attack, or death.[35]

That nagging lack of sleep can literally be killing you. In fact, sleep deprivation has been shown to weaken the immune system, decrease sex drive, increase the risk of diabetes and stroke, worsen mood, diminish the ability to focus, and decrease cognitive performance.[36]

If that's not enough to encourage you to take your sleep seriously, sleep researchers have also found that insomnia often presents in conjunction with an array of psychiatric diseases: depression, anxiety, PTSD, and others.[37] A lack of sleep puts you at risk for other long-term health risks, such as stroke and cardiovascular disease.[38] Sleep loss has even been associated with age-specific increased death.[39]

So, what's the take-away from all these sleep studies? What do they ultimately tell us?

Sleep is vital to our physical and emotional well-being. To understand the value of sleep, we must first get a basic understanding of the biological factors which are present and result in sleep and wakefulness. There are two major determinants of wakefulness: First, our circadian rhythm. The circadian rhythm is the reason for our alertness. It varies based on the time of day.

The second determinant is our homeostatic sleep drive. The homeostatic sleep drive is the reason we have long periods of sleep and can compensate for prolonged wakefulness or strenuous physical activity.

When it comes to the initiation of sleep, melatonin is the key hormone that regulates the sleep/wake cycle. It plays a role in synchronizing the circadian rhythm with the sleep/wake timing. Melatonin is produced by the pineal gland. During the day, the pineal gland is inactive and no melatonin is produced. Once the sun sets and darkness occurs, the pineal gland turns on and produces melatonin. As a result, melatonin levels rise and you feel drowsy and less alert. This results in a desire to sleep. These levels stay elevated in the blood through the night, then fall to low daytime levels once the sun begins to rise. Therefore, light is the dominant factor that controls melatonin. Bright light directly inhibits the release of melatonin. This includes natural and artificial indoor lighting (including lights from artificial devices).

With this basic understanding of how sleep works, the next step is to understand the natural stages of sleep. There are two main types of sleep. One is Non-Rapid Eye Movement sleep (NREM). The other is Rapid Eye Movement sleep (REM). Hang with me for a moment as we take a quick look at the four stages of **NREM sleep**.

Stage 1: Slow rolling eye movements and partial relaxation of voluntary muscles. This is defined as a very light stage of sleep. Usually, this is represented as drowsiness to falling asleep.

Stage 2: On an EEG, this stage is defined by K complexes and spindles. This is a deeper form of sleep (though it is still considered light sleep) with increased relaxation. Our heart rate and body temperature go down during this stage. On average, this stage makes up about 50% of our sleep.

Stage 3 & 4: This is the deepest stage of NREM sleep where growth hormone is released, especially in children. During this stage, it becomes difficult to waken the person and it usually occurs in the first third of the night. Your breathing, blood pressure, and body temperature are further reduced during this stage. This stage is crucial for building up your immune function, repairing injured muscle and tissues, and building up energy for the next day.

REM sleep comprises the smallest portion of your sleep cycle. It occurs several times throughout the sleep cycle during the night. It is characterized by the presence of rapid eye movements and is the deepest stage of sleep. During REM sleep, vivid dreaming occurs. Researchers believe this is important for an individual's memory processing and learning. During REM sleep, you have no motor function and loss of muscle tone. In general, there are 4 to 6 cycles of NREM sleep per night which are followed by brief intervals of REM sleep. Each sleep cycle lasts about 90 minutes. The percentage of REM sleep tends to be highest during infancy and childhood and decreases as you age. The average adult spends about 20-25% of the night in REM sleep. Most REM sleep occurs in the last third of the night, towards the morning.

THE BENEFITS OF SLEEP

B y now, it should be clear that sleep is necessary and essential to your health. In case you need a little more convincing, let's dig a little deeper into the profound benefits of sleep.

While you slumber your body is doing some amazing things. Imagine a team of mechanics working to restore your brain, muscles, and organs. This is especially critical for kids and young adults who are actively growing. Real sleep has numerous benefits, some of which we will touch on here.

There's a flip-side to this pillow. If you're regularly lacking in sleep, deprived of rest, you raise your risk for some chronic health problems. Lack of sleep can have all sorts of negative consequences when it comes to cognitive functions like memory, reaction time, and learning.[40]

Mental and Brain Health

I'm sure we've all been there. We wake up tired, in a fog and shuffle through the motions, to get dressed, and slosh some coffee in a mug, and we somehow find ourselves at work but can't even remember driving our daily route to the office.

A lack of sleep can really tax your brain. Sleep helps your brain work at its best. While you're resting, your brain is getting you ready for the next day. In some ways, it's mending itself from the stresses of the day. For example, new pathways which play a role in learning and remembering information are formed while you sleep.

There's science behind it. Recent studies have shown that a good night's sleep improves learning.[41] Sleep also improves your ability to handle problems big and small. Creativity, decision making, and awareness also improve when you get the proper amount of quality sleep. The opposite is also true. Lacking sleep can lead to a whole host of problems, including causing poor behavior, emotional issues, and even just dealing with everyday life.[42] Talk about an accident waiting to happen. You need good sleep to regulate your mood. Of course, we're sure you already know this. This is evident when you or someone you know isn't that pleasant to be around in the morning. Just think about kids that are tired!

There are even more serious reasons why sleep is so important. Lack of proper sleep has also been shown to lead to an increased risk for depression and even suicide.

This is especially worrying as it's known to be even more of an issue with our youth.[43] Sleep deficient kids are not healthy kids. Lack of sleep in teens and children can cause a myriad of behavior and mental health issues.[44] Sleep deprivation has also demonstrated lower grades and impaired concentration in students.[45] So, get those devices turned off and encourage them to sleep.

The Effects of Sleep on The Body

As we've stated before, sleep aids in healing and repairing your body, especially your heart and blood vessels.[46] Meanwhile, not sleeping well increases your risks for all sorts of health problems like high blood pressure and heart disease to name just a few.[47]

A healthy weight is also influenced by good sleep. Studies have shown that losing sleep increases the chances of becoming obese.[48] You already know that diet and exercise affect sleep, but consider how poor sleep has an effect on weight gain as well as hurts your athletic performance.

When you sleep, your body maintains a healthy balance of hormones. Ghrelin hormones cause a sensation of hunger, whereas leptin gives you that feeling of being full. When you don't get enough sleep, your ghrelin goes up and your leptin goes down. Ever wonder why you crave that midnight snack? Now you know.

Insulin, the hormone that controls your blood sugar level is also affected by lack of sleep, raising your risk of diabetes.[49]

Maybe you think a cat nap every now and then can make up for a lack of nightly sleep. Not so fast. Your body thrives on deep sleep. This is especially true with children and teens. Deep sleep causes hormones to be released in your body that promote normal growth while boosting muscle mass.[50] Deep sleep also helps repair cells and tissues, both in children and adults. Furthermore, research has also shown that sleep plays an important role in puberty and fertility.[51]

Find yourself getting sick often? That packet of vitamin C you dissolve into water may not be the fix you need. You will discover that your immune system needs good sleep to stay healthy. Your immune system will thank you for getting good and regular sleep, and if your immune system is happy, you are much better suited to fight off viruses and other common infections like the dreaded common cold. In fact, research studies have even revealed that sleep can affect the efficiency of vaccinations. Well-rested people who received the flu vaccine developed stronger protection against the illness than those who were sleep-deprived and receiving the same vaccine.[52] When it comes to your health, a good night's rest should be your first line of defense for your immune system, come cold and flu season.

You Wouldn't Want Your Airline Pilot Sleepy, Would You?

We've already covered this fact and it shouldn't come as a surprise: Those who are sleep-deficient are less productive. Whether it's school or work, sleep-deprived people react slower than those who have gotten a good night's sleep. Imagine if you were an airline pilot, charged with the lives of 300 passengers. I'm sure all 300 would want to know that you got a good night's sleep and your reaction time was spot on.

Lack of sleep can also lead to microsleep, those brief moments of sleep that occur when you're normally awake. The danger of microsleep is that it just happens, without your awareness or permission. An example of this would be during a class or a time at work when you don't remember what actually occurred during that brief period of time. Might be harmless in those scenarios, but now imagine that you're a sleepy pilot or even worse a passenger on the sleepy pilot's plane. Sleep deficiency and the microsleep episodes that it can cause can have serious consequences.

Still, many people remain unaware of the dangers of sleep deprivation. Some don't even realize they're sleep deficient. This hazard has been proven out over and over again with everyone from drivers falling asleep at the wheel to boat captains falling asleep at the helm. Sleep deficiency is in many ways as dangerous as being intoxicated while driving. Easily resulting in accidents and even tragic deaths that could have been avoided.

Vehicle accidents aren't the only issue caused by tired people. Whether it's a mistake at work that costs you money or a promotion, a mishap on the factory floor which could result in someone getting seriously injured, or poor performance at school, sleep deficiency can manifest itself in many negative forms. No occasion, endeavor, or occupation is safe from the pitfalls of poor sleep.

And that is why sleep is so important. Sleep helps us think more clearly. It hones our reflexes and sharpens our focus. As sleep researcher Dr. Michael Twery, director of Sleep Medicine, Research and Clinical Research at the National Institute of Health (NIH) put it, "Sleep affects almost every tissue in our bodies. It affects growth and stress hormones, our immune system, appetite, breathing, blood pressure, and cardiovascular health."[53] For your mind, body, and sanity, please take sleep seriously.

CURRENT SLEEP RECOMMENDA-TIONS

By now you may be wondering just how much sleep you should get to stave off all these health risks. Most of us have heard the number eight thrown around. Eight hours of sleep. It's a nice round number. It divides nicely into a 24-hour day, but what do the experts suggest? Let's take a closer look at some of the more current sleep guidelines.

The CDC states that a third of Americans average less than 7 hours of sleep a night. A 2007 study looked at British civil servants who reduced their sleep from 7 to 5 hours or fewer a night. Researchers discovered that they were almost twice as likely to die from all causes (especially cardiovascular disease)[54]. Think about that. If you knew that losing a couple of hours of sleep a night would double your risk of death, would you change your behavior? Would you still give up those sleeping hours to binge watch that show?

You may well ask, how much should I be sleeping? How much should my teenager be sleeping? Recently, the

National Sleep Foundation convened a group of sleep specialists. After their conference, they updated the recommended sleep ranges based on age. Remember, these aren't chiseled-in-stone absolutes. Think of them as recommendations based on a consensus of experts.

We do want to stress the importance of sleep for newborns through young adults. Healthy sleep plays a pivotal role in growth hormone release and development of the brain and body. So, if you're a parent, pay close attention to the recommendations related to your child's age.

Nightly Sleep Recommendations (in hours)

Newborn (0 - 3 months)	14 - 17
Infant (4 - 11months)	12 - 15
Toddler (1 - 2 years)	11 - 14
Preschooler (3 - 5 years)	10 - 13
Children (6 - 13 years)	9 - 11
Teenager (14 - 17 years)	8 - 10
Young Adult (18 - 25 years)	7 - 9
Adult (26 - 64 years)	7 - 9
Older Adults (65+)	7 - 8

SLEEP DISTRACTORS

There are three main distractors that can keep us from sleeping: the body, the mind, and the bed. According to the research of Dr. Rubin Naiman, a pioneer in developing integrative approaches to sleep health, these nightly distractions could be stealing your health. Let's take a closer look at each one of these potential distractors and discover what you can do to mitigate them.

The Physical Body

Our bodies are one of the main culprits that keep us from getting the rest we need. There are two main categories of our bodies that we can focus on: what we eat and our exercise.

Nutrition

To start, food and nutrition play a large role in having successful sleep. Heavy meals should be avoided within 2 - 3 hours of bedtime. We've all had that feeling. You eat a large satisfying meal right before bedtime and when you try to sleep, you're tossing and turning as you feel your body trying to digest your dinner.

Instead, if you must eat prior to sleep to prevent waking up hungry, consider a small night-time snack with a blend of healthy carbs and protein, such as wheat toast with natural peanut butter or chia seeds with bananas. This should prevent any nighttime hunger.

A common question that I am asked is what you should avoid before sleep. There are three common suspects that steal your sleep: caffeine, nicotine, and alcohol.

Caffeine

Caffeine is a stimulant. It's an adenosine receptor antagonist. That means it blocks adenosine from binding to its receptor. Adenosine plays an important role in your sleep/wake cycle. Because caffeine prevents adenosine from binding to its receptor, it prevents you from feeling sleepy. A study from 2013 demonstrated that consuming caffeine 6 hours before bedtime reduced total sleep time by 1 hour.[55] If you love the taste of coffee or tea after dinner, better make it decaf.

Nicotine

Nicotine is also a stimulant. It has been shown to disrupt sleep. Research shows that, compared to non-smokers, smokers spend more time sleeping lightly (Non-REM sleep). Remember, we need the benefit of that deeper REM sleep.

Nicotine has also been shown to change sleep architecture, the stages of your sleep. Multiple studies show smoking has negative effects on overall sleep time, as well as on time spent within each sleep stage.[56] Regular smokers take longer to fall asleep. Overall, they spend less time asleep. Compared to non-smokers, smokers experience less deep sleep. In total, smokers are 4 times more likely to report feeling unrefreshed after a night's sleep than non-smokers. Besides the numerous health advantages, quitting tobacco all together will also improve your overall sleep quality.

Alcohol

It's not uncommon to have a "nightcap" to finish off a meal. According to the National Sleep Foundation, alcohol is the most commonly ingested substance used as a sleep aid. While it may help you fall asleep, it has actually been shown to suppress REM sleep while also increasing the number of awakenings you will have during your sleep as the alcohol wears off. Drinking less is best and preferably with a meal.

In terms of diet, if you suffer from gastroesophageal reflux disease (GERD), try to avoid fatty foods, alcohol, caffeine, and peppermint prior to bedtime. These will make your symptoms worse and possibly prevent you from obtaining good sleep.

When it comes to supporting sleep, magnesium, calcium, and B-Vitamins have been shown to play a role. Before starting any supplements, you should first discuss it with your physician. Our best recommendation would be to avoid caffeine, alcohol, and nicotine six hours before you plan on going to sleep.

EXERCISE

Adequate daytime exercise has been shown to improve sleep. Much has been written regarding the timing of exercise and sleep. Exercise has been shown to decrease stress and it will also "wear you out," both of which promote sleep. Exercising in the early morning or afternoon also helps reset the sleep/wake cycle. Some argue it is best to avoid cardiovascular (aerobic) exercise 3-6 hours prior to sleep. Some believe, due to the elevation in body temperature by exercise, it may interfere with sleep. This doesn't necessarily hold true for everyone. Exercise can affect each individual differently.

If you find yourself very energized by exercise, you may consider exercising earlier in the day. If it wears you out, try it later in the day. As little as 10 minutes of aerobic exercise, such as walking or cycling, can improve the quality of your nighttime sleep. This especially holds true when you exercise on a regular basis.

THE MIND

When we discuss sleep and the mind, we are referring to anxiety, stress, troublesome emotions, and obsessive thoughts. I'm sure you've been there: lying in bed, mind racing, sleep fleeting, or sleep seems almost impossible. Fortunately, there are several simple things you can do to overcome your mind and start easing into a restful sleep.

The first step is mitigating stimulus control. Unfortunately, when we continue to have restless thoughts and are unable to sleep, we begin to associate our bed and bedroom with those sensations. The goal here is to break that cycle and start associating the bedroom with relaxation and sleep. A couple of recommendations to break this cycle are as follows.[57]

1. Go to bed only when feeling sleepy
2. Use your bed only for sleep and sexual activity
3. If you can't sleep, get out of bed and do something relaxing until you feel drowsy, then return to bed

4. Get up at the same time every day even if you haven't slept well

5. Don't nap during the day until nighttime sleep improves

There are also pre-sleep practices you can engage in to help prepare for and promote sleep. These include meditation, guided imagery, muscular relaxation, breathing exercises, and gentle yoga. It's a matter of you finding a method that promotes sleep best for you.

Finally, a personal ritual prior to going to bed is the best way of moving from the waking consciousness to a mental state that supports sleep. Some basic examples are journaling, taking a warm bath, a pre-sleep practice as just mentioned, or an activity you find self-nurturing. Any of these can play a role in calming the mind and helping you get into a state where good sleep is obtainable.

THE ENVIRONMENT

Our environment can have direct effects on our quality of sleep. Ideally, a bedroom should only be used for sleep and sexual activity. The bedroom should be cool, dark, and quiet. Think of it as a relaxing and peaceful space. Not only should it be clean and comfortable, but it should also feel psychologically safe.

The ideal temperature for sleep has been shown to be 68 degrees or less. Additionally, your bedroom should be a quiet environment. If this is not possible, white noise can be implemented by playing nature sounds, or calming music. In some cases, the sound of a speaking voice has been shown to induce sleep.

The mattress and bedding should be comfortable and, ideally, free of any toxins such as pesticides, fire-retardants, or other chemicals. Your mattress and pillow should also provide you with optimal support and comfort.

All clocks should be positioned away from your head. You don't want to be tempted to check the time because this can cause anxiety and promote wakefulness.

Approximately 1-3 hours prior to bedtime, start dimming the lights to help induce melatonin production and a sense of sleepiness.

And finally, for ideal sleep, there should be no use of any device that emits blue light within one hour prior to bedtime. This includes the TV, phone, tablet, or computer. Ideally, there should be no TV in the bedroom. Many sleep-deprived people claim they've sacrificed hours of sleep because of their favorite show.

There are options to purchase blue light glasses, but again, you want to promote the right mental and environmental atmosphere prior to sleep. Reading emails, checking social media, or watching TV doesn't help. On the contrary, those activities can result in a night's worth of ruminative thoughts, resulting in little to no sleep. Our recommandation is to put the electronics outside the bedroom and creating a quiet, dark, peaceful environment that allows you to get the rest you need.

Here is another real-life story to consider.

JB was a female in her 40's who stated she suffered from insomnia. Every night, she attempted to go to bed around 10:30 pm but was unable to fall asleep for at least one to two hours, during which she either just laid in bed or got up and worked on her computer to get a jump on the next day.

She stated she drank coffee but did not have a cup after 3 pm. She stated she did not exercise, nor did she have any specific ritual before bed. She did usually surf on her phone prior to sleep without the use of any blue light blocking eyewear. She also got warm at night but attributed that to just having a warm body.

After some discussion, I made a couple of recommendations. One was to stop looking at any blue screens at least 1 hour before sleep. The other was to decrease the temperature in her bedroom to 68 degrees at night, as this might help her sleep since she noted feeling warm at night.

A daily exercise regimen was also recommended. JB noted she missed yoga and planned to pick back up with her daily practice. It was also suggested she start an evening bedtime ritual, which could include dimming the lights, potentially meditating, or taking a bath before bedtime.

Finally, it was recommended she not just lie in bed at night. Instead, she was to get out of bed and do something besides work, nothing intense, but what would maybe induce sleep. This could include reading a book in a separate room since we would like the bedroom to be associated with sleep.

When I had the chance to follow up with her 2 months later, she stated she had never slept better and she was slowly getting back into shape.

COMMON MYTHS OF SLEEP

The Arizona Center for Integrative Medicine has conducted extensive research into how we sleep, dream, and adapt to sleeplessness. Let's look at some common myths and realities they've discovered about sleep.

Myth: "The mind and body can adapt to less sleep."

Reality: To fully restore itself, the mind and body need to go through all 4 stages of sleep, particularly deep sleep and REM cycles.

Myth: "We should sleep at least 8 hours every night."

Reality: Actually, our personal sleep needs vary with age and other factors. Less than 5 hours can result in health risks. Ideally, we should get between 7-9 hours.

Myth: "It's ideal to always sleep through the night."

Reality: Occasional awakenings are normal.

Myth: "I can and must make myself sleep."

Reality: We can't control the process of falling asleep.

<u>Myth</u>: "I should just stay in bed and rest if I can't sleep."
<u>Reality</u>: It's best to get out of bed at these times.

<u>Myth</u>: "I'll have a terrible day if I don't sleep well."
<u>Reality</u>: Not necessarily. We are very resilient and can adapt to an off night.

<u>Myth</u>: "Good sleepers fall asleep quickly."
<u>Reality</u>: It's normal to take up to 20 minutes to fall asleep.

<u>Myth</u>: "Good sleepers don't dream."
<u>Reality</u>: Dreaming nightly is an essential part of good sleep.

<u>Myth</u>: "It's best to get up and be productive if I can't sleep."
<u>Reality</u>: Being productive at night can disrupt sleep.

<u>Myth</u>: "It's normal to sleep less as we age."
<u>Reality</u>: It's common, but not inevitable, healthy, or normal.

Myth: "It's comforting to check the time when sleepless."

Reality: Clock watching makes it harder to get back to sleep.

In Summary

Hopefully, by now you've discovered some insightful facts about sleep and how it contributes to your health. Let's summarize some key points so you can better prepare yourself for that well-deserved rest.

7 STRATEGIES FOR SLEEP

1) **Ritualize:** Create an energizing ritual with morning light exposure and exercise. Maintain a regular sleep/wake schedule, even on the weekends (don't sleep in for more than 1 or 2 hours). Develop a soothing evening ritual as a bridge to sleep.

2) **Use Dusk and Darkness as Sleep Medicine:** Simulate dusk in your home by dimming the lights for a couple of hours before bed. Always use blue light reduction technology to watch TV or when using computers/phones/tablets. Or even better, avoid using those devices completely before bed. Slow down with a warm bath, journaling, rest practices, yoga, or intimacy. Sleep in total darkness.

3) **Watch Your Diet:** Avoid caffeine, nicotine, sugary foods, and adrenaline prior to sleep. Carefully check

for possible sleep side effects of all medications you use. Check your alcohol intake, drinking less, earlier, and with food.

4) **Quiet your Body Noise:** Keep your bedroom cool (68 degrees or less), dark, and quiet during sleep. Get electric clocks and other such devices away from your head and bedside. Do all you can to feel psychologically safe in your bedroom.

5) **Learn to Surrender to Sleep:** Avoid the chemical knockout of sleeping pills and alcohol. Approach getting to sleep as a personal spiritual practice, an act of faith. Practice "letting go of waking."

6) **Don't Battle Nighttime Wakefulness:** Go to bed only when you feel sleepy. Never watch the clock from bed, it pulls you back into the waking world. If you can't sleep, get up, sit in a comfortable spot until you're sleepy again. Use nighttime wakefulness as an opportunity.

7) **Arise Mindfully with Intention in the Morning:** Obtain at least 20 minutes of daily exposure to morning light shortly after arising. Awaken slowly and explore your grogginess in the morning. Let the memories of your dreams come and note them. Set conscious intentions to guide your waking day. Use these 7 principles to give your body the rest it deserves. Here's to better sleep, a sound mind, and sweet dreams![58]

MOVE

First and foremost: *Please consult your physician before beginning the exercise regimen listed below.*

D
o you remember the movie *Wall-E*©? If you don't, let me give you a quick refresher on this 2008 Disney-Pixar classic. The year is 2805, and due to pollution, humans have abandoned Earth. The story follows a little robot programmed to clean up the filth humanity has left behind, and for reasons unimportant to this particular synopsis, this little robot ultimately ventures into space where humans now reside in a cruise ship-like spacecraft. Earth's former inhabitants are now all obese and move about in a floating chair-like apparatus. All activities are carried out by simply pressing buttons, and no one walks or even moves for that matter, but relies on these floating chairs to get from point A to point B. In this future, people go through life aided by the inventions they've surrounded

themselves with, but ultimately humanity has become a shell of what it used to be.

Although this light-hearted Disney movie intends to be funny, cute, charming, and heartwarming, I found it sobering. I found it sobering because I believe that a technology-assisted, sedentary existence is precisely where we are headed. It also is sobering because, unfortunately, we are currently provided more education on how to interact with technology than we are with how to move our bodies. It is sobering because despite incredible advancements in medicine, we are looking at the first generation in human history to have a shorter life expectancy than their parents.[59] But what if the solution were simple? What if finding the answer depended not on looking to the future, but instead looking backward at the things our ancestors knew. These were what their lives depended on before convenience made existing easy. Specifically, these are the movements that are innate to human function.

This section of *Eat, Sleep, Move, Breathe* focuses on exercise, otherwise known as movement. Our objective is simple: To give you, the reader, practical, applicable exercises you can do to improve your health and well-being, starting today. On the topic of exercise, I like to think in terms of what I call boulders and sand. Boulders are the big, non-negotiable (scientifically backed) aspects of why and what. Sand is the tiny minutia that you will find every pseudo-fitness expert arguing about online. To make our agenda crystal clear, we are here for boulders, not sand.

Before you get turned off by the thought of moving rocks, let me explain that I'm not referring to Stonehenge or loading you up with a three hour per day exercise regimen to follow. There are only three boulders, and I call them Why, What, and How. By that I mean: Why exercise is important; What precisely you need to do; How often, and How to perform these movements and routines safely.

WHY DO I NEED TO BREATHE HARD, LIFT WEIGHTS AND STRETCH?

My three boulders will help build what I like to call "longevity." If you understand these three types of training, why they are essential, and how to properly incorporate them into your exercise regimen, you'll be" cooking with fire," as the saying goes. I mentioned the goal being longevity, which is a concept that's unfamiliar to most. Although many of us understand what fitness or health looks like, most of us rarely consider how health and fitness can affect our freedom. When the aim is longevity, your focus must be on doing that which will support a life unrestricted by the cage, that is immobility. This will reduce your odds of developing the preventable chronic diseases that plague our society. In other words, you want a life free from preventable illness. You want to be able to stand without assistance today, tomorrow, and until the day you pass away. It's that simple.

Let us discuss why you need to breathe hard regularly. Researchers have shown that exercise improves your good cholesterol (HDL) while lowering your bad cholesterol (LDL); strengthens your immune system; increases your lung capacity; decreases levels of depression and anxiety; and these are just some of the numerous benefits. Biomarkers, or in other words, many of those numbers your doctor rattles off when you go for a check-up (blood pressure and resting heart rate being the most common), are also affected positively by regular exercise. This is particularly true about cardiovascular exercise -- exercise that makes you breathe hard for an extended period -- has the unique ability to improve your heart health. If that isn't reason enough to hop on a treadmill and start power walking your way to glory, there has been substantial research in recent years that links this particular type of exercise to significant improvements in mental health, as well.

Fragility in our later years is becoming more and more the norm. As many as 1 in 3 women and 1 in 5 men over 50 years of age will experience an osteoporotic fracture in their lifetime. According to the Stanford Health Care website, "In individuals with osteoporosis, a fracture can be caused by even a minor fall or during routine activities, such as twisting and bending."[60] In numerous studies, strength training has been shown to improve bone density dramatically. Additionally, there is a strong argument to be made that strength is an essential prerequisite for nearly every basic human function. Take walking, standing from a seated position, or simply lifting a glass of water to your mouth; each requires a baseline muscular strength to accomplish. While these are all simple tasks that many take for granted, the weaker you are, the closer you are to losing the necessary strength to perform these tasks.

Conversely, the healthier you are, the further away you are from losing those essential functions, and the more prepared you are for performing more complex tasks like running, jumping, or throwing. The best way to think of this is that you are like a fuel gauge; the stronger you are, the closer you are to full, and the weaker you are, the closer you are to empty. When your gauge is on empty, you can no longer perform many basic human functions unassisted. Consequently, you must hire human help or, like in the movie *Wall-E©*, have machines do those functions for you. When your gauge is full, you not only have the strength to perform these essential human functions with competency, but you also have a solid base for performing other functions not necessary for survival. Instead, these are tasks of choice, like biking, swimming, or more practically, playing a game of tag with your grandchildren.

Let me ask you to try something for me. First, sit on the ground in the crisscross apple sauce style you learned in kindergarten. Then, try to stand without using your hands. Were you able to do this? A study completed in 2012, that surveyed over 2,000 adults, showed that this simple test was a predictor of all-cause mortality.[61] What's the catch, you wonder? There isn't one. It's pretty simple, stronger, more mobile people tend to live longer. Just as mobility is a predictor of longevity, like our discussion on strength, many basic human tasks require a baseline mobility. Take the act of sitting down on the couch for example. When Grandma starts to lose the ability to get down to the couch without falling into it or grabbing another object, family members start to become concerned and start discussing the inevitable move to a nursing home. In contrast, when Grandma can perform a full range of motion squat, family members become more concerned that Grandma's much younger boyfriend may not be able to keep up, rather than finding her a caretaker.

HOW TO TRAIN YOUR CARDI-
ORESPIRATORY SYSTEM

The primary way to train your "cardio," or get you breathing hard as we called it earlier, is through mono-structural movements. These are cyclical movements that can be continuously performed without rest. Think of exercises like running, rowing, biking, swimming, and skiing. Recently, we've experienced a rise in the popularity of Functional Fitness programs (F45, P90x, and Orange Theory) to develop "cardio" by utilizing high repetition gymnastics or light weight lifting to produce the same or similar effect. While those exercises can be very effective too, they carry a high risk if not performed correctly. So, if you're interested in that style of training, our recommendation would be to seek a highly trained coach to teach you the intricacies of the techniques so you can perform those movements safely. By whatever means, your objective is a long, sustainable effort that gets you relatively winded.

The easiest and most scalable of all the "cardio" exercises is running, but what I mean is running at ANY speed. If you're a beginner, walking can be a great way to start. There have been multiple studies citing the efficacy of just increasing the number of steps you take in a day as having a dramatic effect on your overall health. When you start to progress, I encourage you not to go from zero to hero, but instead to go from walking to jogging short distances with walking in between. Gradually build the jogging distances longer with shorter walking distances. As an example, a solid year goal for someone starting with no exercise background would be to finish a 5 kilometer (3.2 miles) run without stopping.

The second exercise I want to touch on is rowing. This is a machine that most people shy away from in the gym because they don't know how to use it properly. I'll try to break it down into a few easy steps, so remember, the mantra I want you to repeat to yourself through the exercise: **"Legs then Arms, Arms then Legs**."

Rowing

1. Set your feet up in the straps; the strap should hit you about midfoot
2. Set the damper (tension on the pull) to 5
3. Grab the paddle with a double overhand grip
4. Drive through your feet until your legs are fully extended
5. Pull until the paddle contacts you at the sternum

6. Extend your arms

7. Bend your legs and return to the start position

Like running, start your rowing slowly and build up your endurance and speed over time. A solid year goal for rowing, coming from an inactive lifestyle, would be to row 10 kilometers without stopping.

Strength Training

Strength can be developed in several ways, but ultimately the methodology comes down to utilizing some form of resistance while performing a movement. To build your strength, you can use traditional weightlifting equipment like barbells, dumbbells, and kettlebells, or perform what we refer to as bodyweight movements. But there is no need to go and purchase expensive equipment or machines immediately. One item I do suggest buying is a lightweight resistance band for its versatility and practicality, especially for those who travel frequently.

To keep strength training simple, we can break exercise down into four categories or muscle groups: core, back, upper body, and lower body.

You will notice that we have included goals for progress after a year of adherence to an exercise program. We want to use these as anchors or targets but to also understand that progress is largely relative. Give yourself the "ok" to progress at whatever pace is reasonable. Never lift or perform something you feel unsafe doing and be proud of every step you take because ultimately its further than you have been before.

Core

The core, for this book's purposes, is defined as the abdominal muscles (six-pack), obliques (meat between your rib cage and hip), and hip flexors (muscles that cross the hip). The reason we start with exercises that primarily target the core is that your success in movements that involve your arms or legs depends heavily on your ability to stabilize your core. The simplest and probably most widely known exercise for your core is the plank position. There are many variations of the plank position, but for our purposes, we will stick with what's called the low plank.

1. Start with your hands together and arms bent
2. Place your forearms on the ground keeping your hands together
3. Straighten your legs out fully behind you

4. Lift your hips and legs from the ground until the only points of contact are your forearms and toes

5. Your body should be in a straight line from the top of your head to the base of your heels

A starting point would be trying to accumulate, over three maximal effort holds, a total of 90 seconds in the low plank position. Someone going from completely inactive to active should set the goal of achieving 2 minutes unbroken after one year of working on this consistently.

Another exercise to add to your repertoire is called the hollow position hold. In explaining this exercise, I will break it down into three separate iterations, beginning level (tuck hold), intermediate level (hollow hold with one leg and one arm extended), and advanced level (full hollow hold).

Beginning Level:
Tuck Hold

If you are aware of a central hernia or diastasis, do not perform this movement, rather, strengthen your core through static isometric contractions, such as the plank, NOT abdominal flexion.

1. Lay down on your back

2. Squeeze your abdominals as though you were performing a crunch, actively pulling the base of your rib cage down toward your belly button

3. At the top of this movement, your hips and shoulders should be lifted slightly from the ground with the middle of your back being the primary point of contact

4. The top position or hold should have your elbows and knees close together with your hips and shoulders lifted off the ground as mentioned before

Intermediate Level:

Hollow Hold with One Arm and Leg Fully Extended

1. Lay down on your back

2. Squeeze your abdominals as though you were performing a crunch, actively pulling the base of your rib cage down toward your belly button

3. Extend one arm overhead while holding the other arm across your chest, extend the opposite leg while pulling the other knee up towards your chest

4. In the final hold position, your shoulders and hips should be mostly off the ground with your lower back being the primary point of contact.

Additionally, your extended arm and leg should hover approximately 1 inch off the ground.

Advanced Level: Full Hollow Hold

1. Lay down on your back
2. Squeeze your abdominals as though you were performing a crunch, actively pulling the base of your rib cage down toward your belly button
3. Extend both arms overhead and extend both legs out fully, pressing your arms and legs together tightly
4. In the hold position, your shoulders and hips should be lifted off the ground, with the primary point of contact being your mid to low back. Your arms and legs should be approximately 1 inch off the ground

Your initial objective when starting this regimen should be to hold a hollow position with a perfect technique for 90 seconds by the end of your first year. Although the low plank and hollow position hold are certainly not an exhaustive list of core exercises, mastering these two will improve your core strength considerably and move you closer to your fitness goals.

Back

The number one thing that people are concerned about when beginning resistance training is injuring their back, and for a good reason. Performing lifts without proper mechanics can lead to catastrophic outcomes. With that in mind, the benefits certainly outweigh the potential risks if lifting is performed correctly. When referring to the back, we are focusing on the spine and the surrounding muscles. The spine is broken down into three basic sections, cervical (neck), thoracic (rib cage and mid-back), and lumbar (lower back). The goal is to strengthen and create awareness in the surrounding muscles on how to simultaneously move and stabilize the spine effectively, or in plain terms, to keep the back safe and get you stronger.

The first exercise I want to cover is called the **sumo deadlift,** due to its transferability to the real world. This movement is essentially the how-to guide on how to pick anything up from the ground to your waist. For that reason, you can use anything to perform it, a backpack, a bag of dog food, one side of a coffee table, or more conventionally a barbell; they all are effective.

1. Straddle the object you are going to pick up in a stance wider than shoulder-width (if this object is a barbell, walk up to it and place the object about midfoot)

2. Imagine your back is a concrete block as you execute the lift, nothing from your head to your hip should move or change position at all.

3. Hinge at the hip until you reach a position similar to an outfielder in baseball

4. Bend the knees by pushing them out but not forward

5. Firmly grasp the object you are lifting

6. Drive through your legs, with your shoulders and hips rising together until the object reaches the knee

7. Push the hips forward to reach a full standing position

Over a year of work, your goal should be to safely lift an object weighing up to your body weight.

The second exercise is called a **Jefferson Curl**; the goal of this exercise is to increase the awareness of how to move each part of your spine independently.

1. Start in a standing position with your feet under your hips

2. Begin by slowly bending your chin towards your chest

3. Follow that by bending the mid-back forward into flexion as well. Go slowly here, vertebrae by

vertebrae. Finally, round the lower-back in the same fashion

4. Finish the movement by extending, vertebrae by vertebrae, back up to a full standing position

As stated in the movement's description, the Jefferson Curl should be performed slowly and unloaded. After a year, you should be able to do this movement up to 20 times without needing to rest between repetitions.

Upper Body

When attempting to improve upper body strength, you will need to target three main areas, pushing, pulling, and small muscle stability. With this goal in mind, I will provide a simple exercise designed to kick start your progress for each area.

Pushing

There are many methods you can use to strengthen your pushing power, but arguably, none are more effective than the overhead press. Specifically, we will discuss the seated dumbbell press. It's important to note that when I say dumbbell, what I mean is two equally weighted objects, and you should not feel limited to using an actual dumbbell.

Kettle-bells or even a couple of milk jugs will do if that's all you have available.

1. Start in a seated position on the ground with your legs extended fully in front of you

2. Bring the dumbbells to your shoulders, with one head of the dumbbell resting on your shoulder with your elbows slightly forward from your hands. This position is what is known as the front rack position

3. Press the dumbbells directly overhead extending your arms fully and reaching up as high as possible to support the weight overhead

4. Maintain a stable and neutral position of your body throughout

5. Finish by bending your elbows forward from your hands and bringing the dumbbells straight back down and returning the dumbbells to the rack position

I encourage anyone reading this book to start with as light weights as possible, develop great technique, and then incrementally increase your load over time. After about a year, a great goal would be to do three sets of 10 with dumbbells totaling a third of your total body weight.

Pulling

For pulling, the **dumbbell row** is a great way to increase your basic strength. Remember, when I say dumbbell, what I mean is two equally weighted objects.

1. Start at a standing position with your arms extended at your waist, grasping the dumbbells
2. Lean forward and hinge at the hip until your torso is close to parallel to the ground (maintain a neutral position of the back)
3. Extend your arms with your palms facing your legs
4. Slowly and deliberately, pull the dumbbells up until they contact you at the base of your rib cage
5. Finish the movement by returning your arms to the fully locked out starting position

As with the overhead press, start light, master the technique, and build slowly. A good year's goal would be to achieve three sets of 10 repetitions with dumbbells totaling one-third of your total body weight.

The last movement, the **banded pull-apart**, is for shoulder stability and targets the small muscles that help keep your shoulders healthy. If you work at a desk and have become increasingly afraid of becoming the Hunchback of Notre Dame, this exercise will be your best friend!

Along with increasing general stability, the banded pull-apart has an extremely restorative effect and can counteract a lot of the negative side effects people experience when sitting at a computer screen for long hours.

1. Using a light tension exercise band (referenced earlier as the ONLY piece of equipment we'd recommend you shell out cash for) grab one side of the band at shoulder width with your palms facing up while holding the band at chest height

2. Pull your hands apart with slow and steady tension until the band contacts your chest

3. Keeping the tension on the band, slowly return your hands to the starting position

A general rule of thumb with strength building is that the most effective movements are often the simplest. Be skeptical if you need to operate 57 pulleys and a lever to perform the movement on some complex machine. That's probably a good indication that that movement will have little to no application in your daily life. A fair year's goal for this simple and effective banded pull-apart is to perform 40 reps without stopping.

Lower Body

Like the upper body, the lower body can be broken down into three basic movement categories: squatting, jumping, and overall lower body stability.

Squatting

We start with the **squat**. Everyone needs to squat, and if you lose the ability to do so, you will struggle to perform common daily tasks like simply sitting and standing. We will talk here about the unloaded squat, but over time the technique discussed here can be used safely to perform a squat under load.

1. Start with your feet shoulder-width apart, and your toes pointed forward

2. Before beginning the squat, brace by taking a deep abdominal breath and squeezing

3. Start by pushing the hips back

4. Bend the knees out so they track in line with your toes

5. Sink into the squat, getting as low as you can and maintaining proper position of the above points. If anything gets out of position, stop an inch higher and work to that range until it's perfect

To reiterate the points above, only go as low as you can maintain proper mechanics. The year goal would be a low (hip crease below the knee) squat maintaining perfect position.

Jumping

The **side-to-side hop** is a wonderful way to increase your balance, coordination, and help with the bone density issue we referenced earlier.

1. Find a crack in the sidewalk or a line on the ground. Preferably, this would be on a firm surface without padding or matting
2. Place both feet together
3. Start by bracing your core, taking a deep abdominal breath and squeezing to stabilize
4. Hop laterally over the line
5. Upon landing, keep your knees in line with your feet and keep your feet together

Note: When you advance, the side-to-side hop can be performed on a single leg as well. At one year, you should look to be able to perform 50 two-footed fluid hops over a line without a break.

Lower Body Stability

The final movement, the **banded sidestep**, targets hip stability and engagement. The hip is arguably the most important joint in lower body function and movement, so strengthening the small stabilizers goes a long way.

1. Take an exercise band and stand at hip distance on one side of the band pulling the remaining side to your waist

2. Take a step with one foot out against the band creating tension

3. Replace the trailing foot to the same width stance as the starting position

4. Perform the same process on the opposite side

In one year, you should shoot to be able to perform 40 reps on each side without taking a break.

IMPROVE YOUR MOBILITY THROUGH STRETCHING

L ike the previous two sections, this will be a simple guide, not an exhaustive list by any means. The aim here will be to give you a few simple stretches that address large areas and multiple muscle groups. Like the strength section, we will break these down into a few categories, core and back, upper body, and lower body.

The core and back are probably the most difficult group of muscles in the body to stretch. While the modified triangle pose that we will cover certainly won't hit every muscle, it goes a long way towards lengthening some of the more difficult and common problem causers.

1. Find a large empty wall space, stand in a straddle stance with your back up against the wall

2. Point one foot forward with the heel up against the wall and the other approximately one foot away from the wall, pointing parallel to the wall

3. Lean from the hip toward the foot running parallel to the wall

4. Keeping your back fully against the wall, reach your arm closest to the foot you are leaning toward and down toward that foot, and the other arm overhead and toward that side, keeping the back of your arms in contact with the wall throughout

5. Repeat on the other side

You should feel this stretch from the top of your hip all the way up to your side and into your shoulder. Your aim should be to hold each side for a minimum of 1 minute without coming out of the stretch.

We talked a bit about the shoulder getting tight from sitting, and especially typing. The prone shoulder stretch will help lengthen the muscles that get short and cause pain.

1. Lay on your stomach

2. Reach one arm out to full extension with your palm down

3. Place your other hand next to your shoulder in the typical pushup position

4. Press into the hand close to your shoulder and rotate your body away from the extended arm until you feel a stretch.

5. Repeat this stretch on the other side

You should feel this stretch in the chest and through the extended arm. You should aim to be able to hold this stretch for 1 minute on each side.

Are you tired of talking about exercise and working out at this point? How about one more, but it will involve a couch. I knew that would work; enter the couch stretch!

1. Take a couch pillow and place it on the ground up against the base of the couch

2. Place your knee on the couch pillow and your foot on the couch

3. Use the ottoman or coffee table to prop your chest up and put your other leg into a modified lunge position

4. Repeat on the other side

You should feel this stretch in your hip and on the front of your leg. Your aim should be to hold this stretch for 1 minute on each side.

Now, the big question is how to take all of this and put it into a plan that you can implement tomorrow. Remember, this is a suggested starting point, but certainly not the only way to do it. What's important is that you start and that you keep going. If you can't handle 3 days, start with 2 or 1, but start and don't stop.

MY TWO-WEEK PROGRAM

(Week One)

WEEK 1: DAY 1	Cardio:	Run or Walk 1 Mile
	Strength:	3 sets each, 10 seated dumbbell press 10 dumbbell rows 40 banded pull apart
	Stretch:	1:00 min triangle stretch (each side) 1:00 min prone shoulder stretch (each side)

WEEK 1: DAY 2	Cardio:	3 x 500-meter row 2:00 min rest between efforts
	Strength:	3 sets each, 1:00 min hollow hold 10 Jefferson curls 1:00 min plank hold 10 deadlifts

	Stretch:	1:00 min triangle stretch (each side) 1:00 min couch stretch (each side)

	Cardio:	3 x 400m run/walk Rest 1:00 min between each 3 x 200m run
WEEK 1: DAY 3	Strength:	60 banded side steps in each direction (in as few sets as possible) Then 5 sets each 10 unloaded squats 20 side to side hops *rest as needed between sets
	Stretch:	1:00 min couch stretch (each side) 1:00 min triangle stretch (each side)

(Week Two)

WEEK 2: DAY 1	Cardio:	row 2000-meters
	Strength:	20 Jefferson curls 4 sets each, 10 deadlifts 10 squats
	Stretch:	1:30 min triangle stretch (each side) 1:30 min couch stretch (each side)

WEEK 2: DAY 2	Cardio:	3 x run/walk 800-meters (rest 6 mins between runs)
	Strength:	4 rounds each, 1:00 min hollow hold Max plank hold Max banded pull aparts
	Stretch:	1:30 min prone shoulder stretch (each side) 1:30 min triangle stretch (each side)

WEEK 2: DAY 3	Cardio:	5 x 200-meter run 250-meter row
	Strength:	Four rounds each, 20 banded side steps (each direction) 12 dumbbell rows 20 side to side hops 12 seated dumbbell press
	Stretch:	1:30 min prone shoulder stretch (each side) 1:30 min triangle stretch (each side) 1:30 min couch stretch (each side)

As you advance on this program, you can increase the difficulty in several ways. First, you may increase the amount of work by adding rounds or repetitions. Second, you could increase the amount of weight or tension of the band. Finally, you can decrease the amount of rest you take between exercises or repetitions.

"Don't be fooled by the calendar. There are only as many days in the year as you make use of. One man gets

only a week's value out of a year while another man gets a
full year's value out of a week." - Charles Richards

The compounding value that even a light amount of regular exercise will have on your health and fitness is incredible. One thing that's important to consider about longevity is that regardless of how healthy we are, no one knows how much longer we have to live. We have absolutely no control of when we pass away because there are so many uncontrollable factors at play. But we do have control over how we live those days and the quality that marks them. With this, we wish the rest of your days be filled with laughter, play, and unrestricted fun. Movement is key, take it seri ously, and you surely won't regret it.

MOVING ON

At 11, SL was already overweight and socially withdrawn. He walked through the doors of our gym with his aunt. She told me SL was a great kid, he just needed something to help him get active. As she was talking, SL stood there with his shoulders slumped. He hunched his back and crossed his arms. He was tall for his age, but by the way he stood, all shelled in, he looked like the smallest kid in the class. I reached out to shake his hand, but could tell he didn't want to be there. The gym was the last place he wanted to be.

Over the next year, SL's routine was to hide in the back of the class and participate as little as possible. He didn't feel like he was fitting in. The less he engaged with the class, the less interest the other kids took in in him.

As a coach, it was hard to watch SL's behavior. He looked like a kid who was going to give up if we couldn't find a way to better engage with him. One day, we decided to talk to his aunt. We thought it'd be a good idea to sign SL up for a lifting meet our gym was hosting. As SL shook his head no in the background, his aunt enrolled him for the meet. SL had regularly attended our lifting classes over the year and had shown great potential. We just needed to get SL to see what we all saw in him.

On the day of the meet, SL was set to compete in the deadlift. As he walked in, he had a particularly grumpy look on his face. Not only was he forced to join the gym and the class, now he was stuck in some stupid competition. When SL started warming up for the deadlift, he looked good, really good. His form looked beautiful. Even though he could easily lift more, the coaches kept the weight light. We didn't want him getting distracted, faltering his technique. When SL trained, he'd do multiple repetitions. But in a weightlifting competition, you only had to perform one rep. And SL's single rep focus was excellent.

For SL's first attempt, he walked onto the platform, with a few people watching, and lifted 265 lbs. with ease. On his second attempt, he lifted 295 lbs. gracefully. Now he had everyone's attention. All eyes were on SL. At 13 years old, he'd already outlifted the next best person by 75 lbs. For SL's final attempt, 315 lbs. were loaded onto the bar. A hush went over the room as SL approached the platform. He grabbed the bar. Pulled flawlessly. And stood tall before the roaring crowd. SL had lifted a personal record by over 100 lbs. That moment changed SL's life.

From then on, he came into the gym with a purpose. He had goals. He had new eating habits. He became more social and outgoing with the other kids. When SL first joined, he was 5'2" and weighed 225. At age 17, he was 6'1" and 205 lbs. That same year he pulled 525 lbs., setting a state record. He's 21 now and SL keeps regular contact with us, the coaches who helped send him on his path.

The one thing that SL's journey made me realize is that confidence isn't built overnight. Instead, it comes from taking step after grueling step up toward what seems like an impossible peak. And before you know it, you can look back at how far you've come, how high you are above where you began. It's then that you realize your goal is closer than when you started. Confidence doesn't come from thinking you can do it. True confidence comes from knowing the effort you've put in and realizing that if you keeping taking the next step there's nothing that can stop you.

Let today become that first step. Put that first foot forward and focus on getting the next foot moving. Then repeat that process over and over. No matter what roadblocks or detours stand in your way, keep your momentum. Keep moving forward. With the will to move, you are an unstoppable force.

Video Links

Plank:
https://www.youtube.com/watch?v=lOI8pKq8mqE&feature=youtu.be

Hollow Hold:
https://www.youtube.com/watch?v=M6Of_X4Qcoo&feature=youtu.be

Sumo Deadlift:
https://www.youtube.com/watch?v=G0FZz7QPIVs&feature=youtu.be

Jefferson Curl:
https://www.youtube.com/watch?v=dfPWUAXKLmg&feature=youtu.be

Seated Press:
https://www.youtube.com/watch?v=e8PWjO-HAZM&feature=youtu.be

Dumbbell Row:
https://www.youtube.com/watch?v=aKdr5drUbFE&feature=youtu.be

Banded Pull Apart:
https://www.youtube.com/watch?v=WnHEXZP6jBE&feature=youtu.be

Air Squat:
https://www.youtube.com/watch?v=EIJdnPKysfw&feature=youtu.be

Side to Side Hop:
https://www.youtube.com/watch?v=ukcb1bUQJHA&feature=youtu.be

Banded Side Steps:
https://www.youtube.com/watch?v=VoM7hO6ycS0&feature=youtu.be

Triangle Pose:
https://www.youtube.com/watch?v=JvZoRHSiD-4&feature=youtu.be

Prone Shoulder Stretch:
https://www.youtube.com/watch?v=rqshJrH8t80&feature=youtu.be

Couch Stretch:
https://www.youtube.com/watch?v=mEfvCsceCds&feature=youtu.be

BREATHE

SP has been isolating at home with her three kids and husband for nine weeks at the time of this writing. Her family noticed she was becoming very irritated and would snap at them for the smallest household infractions. For SP, things were stressful. She felt she had no personal space, no time for herself, and just needed to get away. She loved her family dearly but just needed a break. Unfortunately, that was not much of an option, considering the world situation with the pandemic surrounding her.

When I heard SP's story, it was all too familiar. I recommended that SP start meditating. She should take at least 10-20 minutes, with no distractions, and use a technique. SP found some online meditation guides she could follow and made a rule in her home: When it was her time for meditation, there were to be no disruptions. Soon, her family began seeing a change in SP, particularly with her level of patience and tolerance to the day-in-day-out challenges of parenting three kids. Her family respected her time and would even announce to visitors, *"Be quiet, Mom is meditating."*

Breathe. Technically speaking, breathe is a verb we use for the process of inhaling and exhaling. However, depending upon the context, breathe can be a command to calm down when we're overwhelmed. It can mean to yearn for a sense of freedom as in, "I need a place far away where I can breathe." Also, in what I believe to be its most profound connotation, breathe means to live as in, "As I live and breathe." In this chapter, we'll discuss mindful breathing, the practice of focusing your attention on your breath, the inhale, and the exhale; these are the basics of meditation.

Many people have the wrong perception of meditation. Some think meditation is the exclusive domain of Buddhist monks, or it's tedious and requires a great deal of patience. In fact, meditation does not require believing in any specific religious tradition and, when practiced daily, has many benefits for your physical and psychological well-being. Your daily routine can be spiritual, non-spiritual, formal, or just a very natural way to start caring for yourself. Meditation simply involves incorporating time into your life where your only focus is on you and not the millions of other things which may be of concern to you each day.

We live in a time of constant stimulation. Whether it's our smartphones, the internet, television, or our friends and family, this ongoing struggle for our attention creates stress, and we know that stress can take a toll over time. You may already suffer from a chronic disease or illness which creates even more anxiety. Meditation can help you find peace in a hectic world, but meditation is designed to be a daily practice, and consistency is critical to producing a desirable result.

We recommend starting a formal meditative practice, but if you're not quite there yet, at least consider incorporating some peace into your daily life. This should be a time that's uninterrupted and allows you to escape the world and your thoughts. It can be as simple as sitting in a park and looking at the trees, or sitting quietly in a peaceful place where you can escape all your daily stresses. Where you meditate is up to you, as long as that place provides you some restorative peace. Also, it may help you to know there is no right or wrong when it comes to meditation, it's just what helps you in your daily approach to life, and allows you to re-energize mentally and spiritually.

WHAT IS MEDITATION?

According to the National Center for Complementary and Integrative Health (NCCIH), meditation is "a mind and body practice that has a long history of use for increasing calmness and physical relaxation, improving psychological balance, coping with illness, and enhancing overall health and well-being."[62] Jon Kabat-Zinn, the founder of the University of Massachusetts Center for Mindfulness, describes meditation as "simplicity itself. It's about stopping and being present. That is all."[63]

In a letter published 10 years ago, the director of the NCCIH wrote that "the literature on meditation suggests that it is a potent tool for learning control of attention, regulating emotion, and increasing self-awareness or cultivation of the state called mindfulness."[64] While these insights are well known, within the last 15 years, scientific data have shown that during the practice of meditation there are several measurable biological changes. For example, in the autonomic nervous system, and there is now the recognition that meditation has the potential to have an impact on your mental and physical health. So, even though meditation has been around for centuries, we are just now beginning to understand the positive effects it can have on our health.

In the last 10 years, there has also been quite a bit of focus on Mindfulness, which is actually one aspect of the meditation experience. As defined by Jon Kabat-Zinn, "Mindfulness means paying attention in a particular way; on purpose, in the present moment, and non-judgmentally." The goal of Mindfulness is to have an awareness, moment-by-moment, that disengages you from a strong attachment to beliefs, thoughts, or emotions. The result? Mindfulness creates greater emotional balance, clearer thinking, a heightened sense of compassion, open-heartedness, and well-being. These are all things I believe most of us would like to encompass in our day-to-day living, as well as contributing to a mentally healthy lifestyle.

Why Should I Meditate?

As an individual and a society, we face a daily barrage of stimuli. Many of us suffer from chronic stress, either from psychosocial factors or illnesses which require management tools. As you may know, chronic stress can result in increased levels of cortisol, which alone can result in high blood sugar, hypertension, and fatigue, as well as low-grade levels of inflammation which are associated with an increased risk for disease. Many studies have investigated meditation for different conditions, and there's been growing evidence that it can have multiple health benefits.

Research suggests that meditation can help reduce anxiety and increase positive mental effects. Also, studies have demonstrated that Mindfulness can help prevent recurring depression. In a 1982 study, Jon Kabat-Zinn demonstrated that chronic pain was reduced when the patient was trained in mindfulness-based stress reduction[65]. Studies have also shown that meditation helps with headaches, hypertension, coronary artery disease, overall longevity, cognitive function in older adults, and even quitting smoking.

There have also been numerous studies that demonstrate meditation's role in improving symptoms from psychological disorders, including depression and anxiety, and with individuals who suffer from excessive worry. Given all these findings, meditation has clearly demonstrated a potential benefit for a wide range of disorders, as well as helping you cope with the stresses of daily life.

Health Benefits

One of the primary benefits from meditation appears to be its effect on the autonomic nervous system. This effect results in a decreased sympathetic tone and an increased parasympathetic tone. Have I lost you? Okay, all you need to know is that the sympathetic system becomes more active when you are stressed. It is a part of the "fight or flight" response. As the parasympathetic system is stimulated, however, heart rate and breathing slow, stress hormones decrease, blood vessels dilate, and digestion is facilitated. There have been multiple research studies suggesting meditation can help improve health problems, as well as physically change the brain and body. Gyrification is a brain process in which there is an increase in the folds in the outer layer of the brain. Gyrification was demonstrated in a 2012 study which compared the brain images of 50 adults who meditated and 50 adults who did not meditate. The study suggested that those who meditate have an increase in the folds in the outer layer of the brain which is believed to increase the brain's ability to process information.[66]

Aging is obviously a concern for all of us. We all hope to remain as mentally sharp in our later years as we are in our 20's-30's. A 2013 review of three studies demonstrated the benefits meditation may have on our normal aging process. It noted that meditation may slow, stall, or even reverse changes from the normal aging process in the brain.[67] Meditation has also been postulated to have an effect on our emotions. Our emotions are processed in a part of our brain called the amygdala. In 2012 the NCCIH set out to determine this. It found that different types of meditation can actually affect the amygdala differently, even when the person was not meditating.[68]

Although research is ongoing, past studies have suggested that meditation can help with a wide range of chronic health conditions, including high blood pressure, psychological distress, anxiety, depression, anger, hostility, and coping ability. Recent studies on meditation's ability to reduce pain have produced mixed results. In some studies, scientists suggested that meditation activates certain areas of the brain in response to pain. Even though these studies have demonstrated positive effects of meditation on our brains and internal physiology, there is still a significant amount of research needed to learn the extent of the effect meditation may have on our mind, bodies, and aging process.

Mental Benefits

Like many people, you may be thinking about meditation as a way to manage stress, reduce anxiety, and cultivate peace of mind. There are, however, many studies documenting other lesser-known mindfulness meditation benefits, which can have a positive impact on mental and emotional health. One study from 2014 was a literature review of 47 trials with over 3,000 participants that demonstrated this. It found moderate evidence that mindfulness meditation programs could improve anxiety and depression.[69]

When it comes to research specifically focusing on meditation and anxiety, a review of 36 trials in 2012 found that 25 of them noted the meditation group reported better outcomes for symptoms of anxiety when compared to the non-meditation groups.[70]

It is important to remember that meditation is not meant to replace conventional care, or to be used as a reason to postpone seeing a health care provider about a medical problem.

TYPES OF MEDITATION

If you're ready to take the first steps in starting a daily meditative practice, understand that although there are many types of meditation, most of these have four main elements according to the NCCIH:

1. A quiet location with as few distractions as possible;

2. A specific but comfortable posture (sitting, lying down, walking, or in another position);

3. A focus of attention (a specially chosen word or set of words, an object, or the sensations of the breath); and

4. An open attitude (letting distractions come and go naturally without judging them).

The more common types of meditation include:

- Transcendental Meditation, which uses a mantra
- Mindfulness-based stress reduction
- Zen meditation
- Forest Bathing (yes, it's a type of meditation)
- Kriya Yoga
- Walking meditation
- Forgiveness or Metta meditation

Other practices which incorporate a meditative component include yoga and tai chi. In 2017, the National Health Interview Survey found that some 14.2% of U.S. adults utilized meditation.[71] Those meditative practices often involve a religious context, though many practice meditation without a specific spiritual focus.

Getting Started

Below you will find two simple techniques to start meditating, as well as a mindfulness exercise you can use daily:

The Basics

1. Find a position of comfort. You can either be sitting or lying down. There are meditation chairs and cushions available to purchase for your comfort.

2. Close your eyes.

3. Breathe. Let it naturally flow in and out. Make no effort to control your breath.

4. Focus your attention on your breath without attempting to control its pace or intensity. Pay attention to the movement of your Body as you breathe. This can be as simple as a mental observation of your shoulders, chest, or belly, or watching your breath enter and exit your nose or mouth. If you lose focus or your mind wanders, return your attention back to your breath. Allow thoughts to simply move through you without paying them any particular attention.

When you start to meditate, practice for two to three minutes per day. As you become more comfortable with the practice, begin trying to extend your meditations for longer periods.

Mindfulness Practice

A great way to deal with daily stressors is by also starting a mindfulness practice. This can be done briefly, anywhere, at any time, to help you through the moment. The SOAP mnemonic is a great way to remember the steps and getting started with this practice. [72]

Stop: pause, notice your breathing, and settle into the present moment.

Observe: drop into your body, being aware of and feeling whatever is happening at this moment.

Assess: without judgment, recognize the pleasant, unpleasant, neutral nature of this experience and let it go.

Proceed: take a deep breath and move on.

WALKING MEDITATION

The steps below are adapted from a guided walking meditation led by Kabat-Zinn's (2014) *Mindfulness Meditation in Everyday Life and Exercises and Meditations.* [73]
The time required to complete a walking meditation is about 10 minutes.

First: find a location where you can walk about 10-15 paces back and forth. It should be a quiet place where you won't be disturbed. It can be indoors or outdoors, wherever you feel the most comfortable.

Second: walk along the path you chose while stopping to breathe for as long as you like before returning in the opposite direction. You should pause and breathe at the end of your steps just before turning around. The goal of walking meditation is to think about walking, which you normally do automatically. You should try to focus on the 4 components of each step:

1. Lifting one foot;

2. Moving the foot a bit forward from where you're standing;

3. Placing the heel of the foot on the floor first, followed by the rest of the foot;

4. Shifting your body weight onto the forward leg as the back-heel lifts while the toes of the foot remain touching the ground;

5. Lifting the back foot entirely off the ground;

6. Observing the back foot as it swings forward and lowers;

7. Paying attention to the back foot as it makes contact with the ground, heel first; and

8. Feeling the weight shift onto that foot as the body moves forward.

When it comes to speed, walking meditation should be a slow process that involves taking small, deliberate steps.

They should feel natural and not exaggerated. Your hands can be clasped together in front or behind you, or just have them hanging at your side, whatever feels comfortable for you.

Third: Your attention should be focused on the sensations you usually take for granted while you are taking steps, such as your breath coming in and going out of your body; the feeling of moving your feet and legs as they touch the ground and move forward; the sensation of your head, neck, shoulders, and back as you utilize them in balancing your body for each step; sounds around you as you take the steps, either from you or from the steps themselves; and finally, whatever your eyes focus on as you are moving across the ground. The goal is to fix your attention on any one of these sensations. If your mind wanders (which it will in the beginning), it's okay. Just notice it wandering and then refocus on one of the sensations.

The more you practice your particular meditation technique, the more it will bring mindfulness into the rest of your life. You may notice a sense of peace or awareness in other activities you perform. Above all, remember your daily meditation practice is your time. Protect it at all costs and enjoy the peace it can provide. In closing, the following case demonstrates how meditation can be applied to help deal with life's challenges.

CG was a successful male in his 30's. He was a good friend who had made multiple visits to the ER for chest tightness and palpitations. Each time, he stated he was convinced he was having a heart attack. He had multiple stress tests and visits to the cardiologist, all of whom stated his heart was fine and he was more likely suffering from anxiety.

It took some time, but CG finally began accepting the fact that maybe it was anxiety. He did note he had a very stressful job and family situation, but otherwise he had no cardiac risk factors, exercised daily, and ate a mostly vegetarian diet.

When he approached me about what to do, I asked him some basic lifestyle questions and encouraged him to continue to exercise as it would also help alleviate some of the stress he may have been experiencing.

When I suggested professional help, he expressed that he never wanted to be on any medications and refused to see a psychiatrist or psychologist to discuss some of his personal issues; he felt he could handle them on his own. With this being said, I decided to suggest guided meditations for him to perform daily in an attempt to alleviate his stress. I also suggested a specific breathing technique if he were to have a panic attack. CG initially rolled his eyes and stated,

"I knew you would suggest something like that."

Even though he was reluctant, he started a daily meditative practice, which started with 5 minutes each morning and each night. Little did I know that 5 minutes became 30 minutes twice a day. CG noted he felt calmer than he had in years, though he would still have episodes here and there. During episodes, he would either meditate or perform the breathing technique which appeared to help. He also noted he was now considering speaking to a professional, as he felt he had a better grasp of what may be triggering his anxiety.

WELL DONE!

Congratulations! You've not only finished the book, but you're also on your way to starting a new chapter in life. One where you're eating cleaner, feeling rested, having a spring in your step, and maintaining a sounder mind. With a basic understanding of our four pillars of health: Eat, Sleep, Move, Breathe, you have the foundation to build a stronger, healthier you. As you build your future, we'd like to leave you with one last word of encouragement.

What you're practicing is not a diet or exercise routine. Think of it as a new way of life. Like putting on your seatbelt, or tying your shoes, think of these pillars as foundational items that you just do. Make this new way of life more than a habit, make it part of your life.

As you do this, stay positive. The road to a healthier you is full of stress, temptations, and battles. You may not always win each day, but keep positive. Remember to forgive yourself and stay resilient. Each choice you make, each step you take toward your health, however small, makes a difference.

So why not today? Why not let this day be the start of your journey? You can have a body, mind, and lifestyle that you love but it starts with you making a choice to begin. It starts with a single step. We encourage you to let today be the start of your good health and happiness.

Thank you for letting us be a part of this journey. Here's to a better, stronger you. We salute you: To your health!

ABOUT THE AUTHORS

Dr. Lars Thestrup, MD.
Dr. Lars Thestrup was born and raised in Northern Virginia where he attended Mary Washington College earning his B.S. in Biology. He received his M.D. at the Medical College of Virginia and completed his emergency medicine residency at Johns Hopkins. Lars then completed a fellowship in North Carolina, focusing on emergency medical services and disaster preparedness at the Carolinas Medical Center. Shortly after the completion of his fellowship, he accepted a position in the City of Houston where he currently serves as an EMS Physician and practices at several emergency departments. Over time he realized his passion for health and fitness and its role in the prevention of disease which subsequently led him to the University of Arizona Integrative Medicine Fellowship. This has allowed him to continue his journey in helping others evaluate their current lifestyles and assist them in obtaining their individual goals. This book is an extension of that passion which he hopes will transform and

educate those truly looking for a change. When he is not working, he loves to spend time outdoors with his wife and two kids.

Jennifer Pfleghaar, DO, FACEP, ABOIM.

Dr. Jennifer Pfleghaar was born and raised in Erie, PA. She attended undergraduate at Kent State University with a B.S. in Zoology/Pre-Med and went back to her hometown for medical school at Lake Erie College of Osteopathic Medicine. Dr. Pfleghaar completed her Emergency Medicine residency at St. Vincent Mercy Medical Center in Toledo, OH and a 2-year fellowship in Integrative Medicine at the University of Arizona. She works in local community Emergency Rooms around Toledo, OH. She is double board certified in Emergency Medicine and Integrative Medicine. Dr. Pfleghaar is the owner of PflegMed: Center for Integrative Medicine and Natural Aesthetics and Perrysburg Yoga where she sees patients and teaches yoga. Her own health dilemma of Hashimoto's disease, having MTHFR mutations and having her own children made her journey into Integrative Medicine a passion and a way of life. She lives in Toledo with her husband Chip and four children which keep her very busy! They enjoy making gluten/dairy free desserts together and chasing around their backyard chickens.

Connor Martin was born in San Diego, California to parents Jeff and Mikki Martin, founders of The Brand X Method, an internationally recognized youth strength and conditioning program. He grew up steeped in the fitness world and is fondly referred to as the "crash test dummy." He is also widely known within the functional fitness community as the original kid participating in this style of exercise. Connor spent his first few adult years as a seminar staff member for CrossFit Inc., teaching the Level 1, Level 2, and CrossFit Kids Seminars to aspiring CrossFit trainers. At the age of 24, Connor moved his young family to Houston, Texas and assumed the head coaching position at CrossFit EaDo, and later also CrossFit Central Houston. Connor is now a lead coach at P3 CrossFit, owns an online fitness company, Compete Elite, and is the International Training Center coordinator for The Brand X Method. He resides in Houston with his fiancé Michelle and their three children.

ABOUT
KHARIS PUBLISHING

KHARIS PUBLISHING is an independent, traditional publishing house with a core mission to publish impactful books, and channel proceeds into establishing mini-libraries or resource centers for orphanages in developing countries, so these kids will learn to read, dream, and grow. Every time you purchase a book from Kharis Publishing or partner as an author, you are helping give these kids an amazing opportunity to read, dream, and grow. Kharis Publishing is an imprint of Kharis Media LLC. Learn more at https://www.kharispublishing.com.

REFERENCES

EAT

[1] Proc Nutr Soc. 2010 Aug;69(3):273-8. doi: 10.1017/S002966511000162X. Epub 2010 Jun 2. Flavonoids as anti-inflammatory agents.Serafini M1, Peluso I, Raguzzini A. Add in 2 Webb AL, McCullough ML. Dietary lignans: potential role in cancer prevention. Nutr Cancer. 2005;51(2):117-31. doi: 10.1207/s15327914nc5102_1. PMID: 15860433.

[2] Manheimer EW, van Zuuren EJ, Fedorowicz Z, Pijl H. Paleolithic nutrition for metabolic syndrome: systematic review and meta-analysis. Am. J. Clin. Nutr. 102(4):922-32Oct, 2015

[3] Am J Clin Nutr. 1982 Nov;36(5):873-7. Vegetarianism, dietary fiber, and mortality. Burr ML, Sweetnam PM

[4] O SS, Yu S, Fedewa A. Systematic review: dietary fibre and FODMAP-restricted diet in the management of constipation and irritable bowel syndrome. Aliment. Pharmacol. Ther. 41(12):1256-70 Jun, 2015

[5] Inflamm Bowel Dis. 2017 Nov.; 23(11):2054-2060. doi: 10.1097/MIB.0000000000001221.

Efficacy of the Autoimmune Protocol Diet for Inflammatory Bowel Disease. Konijeti GG1, Kim N, Lewis JD, Groven S, Chandrasekaran A, Grandhe S, Diamant C, Singh E, Oliveira G, Wang X, Molparia B, Torkamani A.

[6] Cureus. 2019 Apr 27;11(4): e4556. doi: 10.7759/cureus.4556.Efficacy of the Autoimmune Protocol Diet as Part of a Multi-disciplinary, Supported Lifestyle Intervention for Hashimoto's Thyroiditis. Abbott RD1, Sadowski A2, Alt AG3.

[7] Arch Latinoam Nutr. 2008 Dec;58(4):323-9. [Ketogenic diets: additional benefits to the weight loss and unfounded secondary effects].

[8] Müller II, de Toledo FW, Resch KL. Fasting followed by vegetarian diet in patients with rheumatoid arthritis: a systematic review. *Scand J Rheumatol.* 2001;30(1):1-10. doi:10.1080/030097401750065256

[9] Pak J Biol Sci. 2012 Mar 1;15(5):255-8. Effect of fasting with two meals on BMI and inflammatory markers of metabolic syndrome. Shariatpanahi MV1, Shariatpanahi ZV, Shahbazi S, Moshtaqi M.

[10] J Pain. 2016 Mar;17(3):275-81. doi: 10.1016/j.jpain.2015.11.002. Epub 2016 Feb 2. Increasing Neuroplasticity to Bolster Chronic Pain Treatment: A Role for Intermittent Fasting and Glucose Administration? Sibille KT1, Bartsch F2, Reddy D3, Fillingim RB3, Keil A4

[11] Rowe KS, Rowe KJ. Synthetic food coloring and behavior: a dose response effect in a double-blind, placebo-controlled, repeated-measures study. J Pediatr. 1994;125(5 Pt 1):691-698. doi:10.1016/s0022-3476(94)70059-1

[12,] Arnold LE, Lofthouse N, Hurt E. Artificial food colors and attention-deficit/hyperactivity symptoms: conclusions to dye for. Neurotherapeutics. 2012;9(3):599–609. doi:10.1007/s13311-012-0133-x

[13] Stevens LJ, Burgess JR, Stochelski MA, Kuczek T. Amounts of artifical food colors in commonly consumed beverages and potential behavioral implications for consumption in children. Clin Pediatr (Phila). 2014 Feb;53(2):133-40. dio: 10.1177/0009922813502849. Epub 2013 Sep 13. PMID: 24037921.

[14] Boris M, Mandel FS. Foods and additives are common causes of the attention deficit hyperactive disorder in children. Ann Allergy. 1994;72(5):462-468.

[15] The consumption of added sugars (caloric sweeteners) has been linked to obesity, diabetes, and heart disease) Welsh JA, Sharma AJ, Grellinger L, Vos MB. Consumption of added sugars is decreasing in the United States. Am. J. Clin. Nutr. 94(3):726-34 Sep, 2011

[16] Joyner, M. A., Gearhardt, A. N., & White, M. A. (2015). Food craving as a mediator between addictive-like eating and problematic eating outcomes. Eating behaviors, 19, 98–101. https://doi.org/10.1016/j.eatbeh.2015.07.005

[17] Freeman CR, Zehra A, Ramirez V, Wiers CE, Volkow ND, Wang GJ. Impact of sugar on the body, brain, and behavior. Front Biosci (Landmark Ed). 2018;23:2255-2266. Published 2018 Jun

[18] Ahmed SH, Guillem K, Vandaele Y. Sugar addiction: pushing the drug-sugar analogy to the limit. Curr Opin Clin Nutr Metab Care. 2013;16(4):434-439. doi:10.1097/MCO.0b013e328361c8b8

[19] Lenoir M, Serre F, Cantin L, Ahmed SH. Intense sweetness surpasses cocaine reward. PLoS One. 2007;2(8): e698. Published 2007 Aug 1. doi:10.1371/journal. pone.0000698

[20] Science. 2019 Mar 22;363(6433):1345-1349. doi: 10.1126/science.aat8515.

High-fructose corn syrup enhances intestinal tumor growth in mice. Goncalves MD1,2, Lu C3, Tutnauer J1, Hartman TE4, Hwang SK1, Murphy CJ1,5, Pauli C6, Morris R4, Taylor S1, Bosch K7, Yang S8, Wang Y8, Van Riper J8, Lekaye HC9, Roper J10, Kim Y11, Chen Q3, Gross SS3, Rhee KY4, Cantley LC12, Yun J13.

[21] Am J Clin Nutr. 2014 Sep;100(3):833-49. doi: 10.3945/ajcn.114.086314. Epub 2014 Aug 6. Fructose, high-fructose corn syrup, sucrose, and nonalcoholic fatty liver disease or indexes of liver health: a systematic review and meta-analysis. Chung M1, Ma J1, Patel K1, Berger S1, Lau J1, Lichtenstein AH1.

[22] Am J Clin Nutr. 2012 Feb;95(2):283-9. doi: 10.3945/ajcn.111.022533. Epub 2011 Dec 28. Sucrose-sweetened beverages increase fat storage in the liver, muscle, and visceral fat depot: a 6-mo randomized intervention study. Maersk M1, Belza A, Stødkilde-Jørgensen H, Ringgaard S, Chabanova E, Thomsen H, Pedersen SB, Astrup A, Richelsen B.

[23] BMJ. 2008 Feb 9;336(7639):309-12. doi:

10.1136/bmj.39449.819271.BE. Epub 2008 Jan 31. Soft drinks, fructose consumption, and the risk of gout in men: prospective cohort study. Choi HK, Curhan G. Soft drinks, fructose consumption, and the risk of gout in men: prospective cohort study. BMJ. 2008 Feb 9;336(7639):309-12. doi: 10.1136/bmj.39449.819271.BE. Epub 2008 Jan 31. PMID: 18244959; PMCID: PMC2234536.

[24] Front Biosci (Landmark Ed). 2018 Jun 1;23:2255-2266. Impact of sugar on the body, brain, and behavior. Freeman CR1, Zehra A1, Ramirez V1, Wiers CE2, Volkow ND2, Wang GJ3.

[25] Curr Gastroenterol Rep. 2017 Nov 21;19(12):64. doi: 10.1007/s11894-017-0602-9. The Association Between Artificial Sweeteners and Obesity. Pearlman M1, Obert J2, Casey L3.

[26] Lippi G, Franchini M, Favaloro EJ, Targher G. Moderate red wine consumption and cardiovascular disease risk: beyond the "French paradox". *Semin Thromb Hemost.* 2010;36(1):59-70. doi:10.1055/s-0030-1248725

[27] Adv Exp Med Biol. 2017 ; 956 :61-84. doi: 10.1007/5584_2016_147. Impact of Salt Intake on the Pathogenesis and Treatment of Hypertension. Rust P1, Ekmekcioglu C2.

[28] Mayo Clin Proc. 2013 Sep;88(9):987-95. doi: 10.1016/j.mayocp.2013.06.005. Role of dietary salt and

potassium intake in cardiovascular health and disease: a review of the evidence. Aaron KJ1, Sanders PW.

[29] Poonamjot Deol, Elena Kozlova, Matthew Valdez, Catherine Ho, Ei-Wen Yang, Holly Richardson, Gwendolyn Gonzalez, Edward Truong, Jack Reid, Joseph Valdez, Jonathan R Deans, Jose Martinez-Lomeli, Jane R Evans, Tao Jiang, Frances M Sladek, Margarita C Curras-Collazo, Dysregulation of Hypothalamic Gene Expression and the Oxytocinergic System by Soybean Oil Diets in Male Mice, Endocrinology,bqz044, https://doi.org/10.1210/endocr/bqz044 Sibille KT1, Bartsch F2, Reddy D3, Fillingim RB3, Keil A4.

SLEEP

[30] Morris, C. J., Aeschbach D., & Scheer F. A. (2012). Circadian system, sleep and endocrinology. Mol. Cell. *Endocrinolo.*;349;91-104.)

[31] Ancoli-Israel S., & Rot, T. (1999). Characteristics of insomnia in the united states: Results of the 1991 National Sleep Foundation Survey. I. *Sleep.* 22(Suppl 2): S347-53.

[32] Lozoff, B, Wolf, AW, and Davis, NS. Sleep problems seen in pediat- ric practice. Pediatrics 1985;75:477-483.

Armstrong, KL, Quinn, RA, and Dadds, MR. The sleep patterns of normal children. Med J Aust 1994;161:202-206.

Burnham, MM, Goodlin-Jones, BL, Gaylor, EE, and Anders, TF. Nighttime sleep-wake patterns and self-soothing from birth to one year of age: a longitudinal intervention study. J Child Psychol Psy- chiatry 2002;43:713-725.

Goodlin-Jones, BL, Burnham, MM, Gaylor, EE, and Anders, TF. Night waking, sleep-wake organization, and self-soothing in the first year of life. J Dev Behav Pediatr

2001;22:226-233.

Mindell, JA. Empirically supported treatments in pediatric psychol- ogy: Bedtime refusal and night wakings in young children. Journal of Pediatric Psychology 1999;24:465-481.

Bixler, EO, Kales, JD, Scharf, MB, Kales, A, and Leo, LA. Inci- dence of sleep disorders in medical practice: A physician survey. Sleep Research 1976;5:62.

Mindell, JA, and Durand, VM. Treatment of childhood sleep disor- ders: Generalization across disorders and effects on family mem- bers. Special issue: Interventions in pediatric psychology. J Ped Psychol 1993;18:731-750.

Byars KC, Yolton K, Rausch J, Lanphear B, Beebe DW. Prevalence, patterns, and persistence of sleep problems in the first 3 years of life. Pediatrics 129(2):e276-84 Feb, 2012

[33] National Sleep Foundation's Inaugural Sleep Health Index™. (2014). Sleepfoundation.org

[34] University of Pennsylvania School of Medicine. (2018, June 5). One in four Americans develop insomnia each year: 75 percent of those with insomnia recover. *ScienceDaily*. Retrieved August 7, 2020 from www.sciencedaily.com/releases/2018/06/180605154114.htm

[35] Phillips B, Mannino DM. Do insomnia complaints cause hypertension or cardiovascular disease? J Clin Sleep Med 3(5):489-94 15 Aug, 2007.

[36] Institute of Medicine (US) Committee on Sleep Medicine and Research; Colten HR, Altevogt BM, editors. Sleep Disorders and Sleep Deprivation: An Unmet Public Health Problem. Washington (DC): National Academies Press (US); 2006. 3, Extent and Health Consequences of Chronic Sleep Loss and Sleep Disorders.

[37] Zimmerman M, McGlinchey JB, Young D, Chelminski I.

Diagnosing major depressive disorder I: A psychometric evaluation of the DSM-IV symptom criteria. *J Nerv Ment Dis* 2006;194:158–163.

Schwartz DJ, Kohler WC, Karatinos G. Symptoms of depression in individuals with obstructive sleep apnea may be amenable to treatment with continuous positive airway pressure. *Chest* 2005;128:1304–1306.

Alfano, C. A., & Gamble, A. L. (2009). The Role of Sleep in Childhood Psychiatric Disorders. *Child & youth care forum*, *38*(6), 327–340. https://doi.org/10.1007/s10566-009-9081-y

[38] Yaggi HK, Concato J, Kernan WN, Lichtman JH, Mohsenin V. Obstructive Sleep apnea as a risk factor for stroke and death. NEJM 2005;353(19):2034-2041.

Bradley TD, Logan AG, Kimoff RJ, Series F, Morrison D, Ferguson K, Belenkie I, Pfeifer M, Fleetham J, Hanly P, Smilovitch M, Tomlinson G, Floras JS. Continuous positive airway pressure for central sleep apnea and heart failure. NEJM. 2005;353(19):2025-2033.

Caples SM, Gami AS, Somers VK. Obstructive sleep apnea. Annals of Internal Medicine. 20015;142(3):187-197.

Liu Y, Tanaka H. Fukuoka Heart Study Group. Overtime work, insufficient sleep, and risk of non-fatal acute myocardial infarction in Japanese men. Occupational and Environmental Medicine. 2002;59(7):447-451.

Ayas NT, White DP, Manson JE, Stampfer MJ, Speizer FE., Malhotra A, Hu FB. A prospective study of sleep duration and coronary heart disease in women. Archives of Internal Medicine. 2003;163(2):205-209.

[39] Kripke DF, Garfinkel L, Wingard DL, Klauber MR,

Marler MR. Mortality associated with sleep duration and insomnia. Archives in General Psychiatry. 2002;59(2):131-136.

Tamakoshi A, Ohno Y. JACC Study Group. Self-reported sleep duration as a predictor of all-cause mortality: Results from the JACC study, Japan. Sleep. 2004;27(1):51-54.

Patel SR, Ayas NT, Malhotra MR, White DP, Schernhammer ES, Speizer FE, Stampfer MJ, Hu FB. A prospective study of sleep duration and mortality risk in women. Sleep. 2004;27(3):440-444.

[40] Waterhouse, J. Circadian Rhytms in Cognition. Progress in Brain Research. 2010;185:131-153.

Frenda S,F enn, KM. Sleep less, think worse: The effect of sleep deprivation on working memory. Journal of applied Research in Memory and Cognition. 2016;5(4):463-469.

Alhola, P., & Polo-Kantola, P. (2007). Sleep deprivation: Impact on cognitive performance. *Neuropsychiatric disease and treatment*, *3*(5), 553–567.

[41] *Maria Bagby (25 February 2014). "The Role of Sleep in Memory, Learning, and Health". Therapeutic Literacy Center. Retrieved 29 September 2018.* "To understand the big picture, give it time – and sleep". *EurekAlert.* 20 April 2007. Retrieved 23 April 2007.

Tononi, Giulio; Cirelli, Chiara (1 January 2006). "Sleep function and synaptic homeostasis". *Sleep Medicine Reviews.* **10** (1):49–62. doi:10.1016/j.smrv.2005.05.002. Graves L, Pack A, Abel T. Sleep and memory: a molecular perspective. Trends Neurosci. 2001;24:237–43. [PubMed] [Google Scholar]

Maquet P. The role of sleep in learning and

memory. Science. 2001;294:1048–52[PubMed] [Google Scholar]. Stickgold R. Sleep-dependent memory consolidation. Nature. 2005;437:1272–8.

[PubMed] [Google Scholar].

Ellenbogen JM, Hulbert JC, Stickgold R, Dinges DF, Thompson-Schill SL. Interfering with theories of sleep and memory: sleep, declarative memory, and associative interference. Curr Biol. 2006;16:1290–4.[PubMed] [Google Scholar].

Walker MP, Stickgold R. Sleep, memory, and plasticity. Annu Rev Psychol. 2006;57:139–66.

Killgore WDS. Effects of sleep deprivation on cognition. Prog Brain Res 185: 105–129, 2010

42 Watling J, Pawlik B, Scott K, Booth S, Short MA. Sleep loss and affective functioning: more than just mood. Behav Sleep Med. 2017;15(5):394–409. doi: 10.1080/15402002.2016.1141770.

Brown LK. Can sleep deprivation studies explain why human adults sleep? Curr Opin Pulm Med 18: 541–545, 2012.

Vandekerckhove M, Cluydts R. The emotional brain and sleep: an intimate relationship. Sleep Med Rev 14: 219–226, 2010 [PubMed] [Google Scholar]

43 Zimmerman M, McGlinchey JB, Young D, Chelminski I. Diagnosing major depressive disorder I: A psychometric evaluation of the DSM-IV symptom criteria. *J Nerv Ment Dis* 2006;194:158–163.

Schwartz DJ, Kohler WC, Karatinos G. Symptoms of depression in individuals with obstructive sleep apnea may be amenable to treatment with continuous positive airway pressure. *Chest* 2005;128:1304–1306.

Fawcett J, Scheftner WA, Fogg L, Clark DC, Young MA, Hedeker D, Gibbons R. Time-related predictors of suicide in major affective disorder. Am J Psychiatry. 1990 Sep;147(9):1189–94. doi: 10.1176/ajp.147.9.1189. [PubMed] [CrossRef] [Google Scholar]

Ağargün MY, Kara H, Solmaz M. Sleep disturbances and suicidal behavior in patients with major depression. J Clin Psychiatry. 1997Jun;58(6):249–51. [PubMed] [Google Scholar]

Turvey CL, Conwell Y, Jones MP, Phillips C, Simonsick E, Pearson JL, Wallace R. Risk factors for late-life suicide: a prospective, community-based study. Am J Geriatr Psychiatry. 2002;10(4):398–406.

[44] Cara A. Palmer, Candice A. Alfano. **Sleep and emotion regulation: An organizing, integrative review.** *Sleep Medicine Reviews*, 2016; DOI: 10.1016/j.smrv.2015.12.006

[45] Roth, Daphne Ari-Even; Kishon-Rabin, Liat; Hildesheimer, Minka; Karni, Avi (1 February 2005). "A latent consolidation phase in auditory identification learning: Time in the awake state is sufficient". *Learning & Memory*. **12** (2): 159–164.

[46] McAlpine, C.S., Kiss, M.G., Rattik, S. *et al.*Sleep modulates haematopoiesis and protects against atherosclerosis. *Nature* 566, 383–387 (2019).

[47] Kasasbeh E, Chi DS, Krishnaswamy G. Inflammatory aspects of sleep apnea and their cardiovascular consequences. *South Med J*2006;99:58–67.

Calhoun DA, Harding SM. Sleep and Hypertension. CHEST 2010;138(2)434-43.

[48] Beccuti, G., & Pannain, S. (2011). Sleep and

obesity. *Current opinion in clinical nutrition and metabolic care*, *14*(4), 402–412.

Taheri S. The link between short sleep duration and obesity: We should recommend more sleep to prevent obesity. *Arch Dis Child* 2006;91:881–884.

Morselli L, Leproult R, Balbo M, Spiegel K. Role of sleep duration in the regulation of glucose metabolism and appetite. Best Pract Res Clin Endocrinol Metab. 2010;24:687–702.[PMC free article] [PubMed] [Google Scholar]

Knutson KL. Sleep duration and cardiometabolic risk: a review of the epidemiologic evidence. Best Pract Res Clin Endocrinol Metab. 2010;24:731–743.

[49] Mesarwi, O., Polak, J., Jun, J., & Polotsky, V. Y. (2013). Sleep disorders and the development of insulin resistance and obesity. *Endocrinology and metabolism clinics of North America*, *42*(3), 617–634.

Beccuti, G., & Pannain, S. (2011). Sleep and obesity. *Current opinion in clinical nutrition and metabolic care*, *14*(4), 402–412.

Gottlieb DJ, Punjabi NM, Newman AB, Resnick HE, Redline S, Baldwin CM, Nieto FJ. Association of sleep time with diabetes mellitus and impaired glucose tolerance. Archives of Internal Medicine. 2005;165(8):863-867.

Knutson KL, Ryden AM, Mander VA, Van Cauter E. Role of sleep duration and quality in the risk and severity of type 2 diabetes mellitus. *Arch Intern Med* 2006;166:1768–1764.

[50] Ritsche, K., Nindl, B. C., & Wideman, L. (2014). Exercise-Induced growth hormone during acute sleep deprivation. *Physiological reports*, *2*(10), e12166.

[51] Lateef, O. M., & Akintubosun, M. O. (2020). Sleep and Reproductive Health. *Journal of circadian rhythms*, *18*,

1. https://doi.org/10.5334/jcr.190

N. D. Shaw, J. P. Butler, S. M. McKinney, S. A. Nelson, J. M. Ellenbogen, J. E. Hall. **Insights into Puberty: The Relationship between Sleep Stages and Pulsatile LH Secretion**. *Journal of Clinical Endocrinology & Metabolism*, 2012; DOI: 10.1210/jc.2012-2692

[52] Taylor, D. J., Kelly, K., Kohut, M. L., & Song, K. S. Is Insomnia a Risk Factor for Decreased Influenza Vaccine Response?. *Behavioral sleep medicine*,2017; *15*(4), 270–287.

Spiegel K, Sheridan, JF, Van Cauter, E. Effect of Sleep Deprivation on Response to Immunization. JAMA. 2002;288(12)1471-1472

[53] The Benefits of Slumber. NIH News in Health. https://newsinhealth.nih.gov/2013/04/benefits-slumber. April 2013.

[54] Ferrie J, Shipley M, Cappuccio F, Bruner E, Miller M, Kumari M, Marmot M. A Prospective Study of Change in Sleep Duration: Associations with Mortality in the Whitehall II Cohort. Sleep. 2007;30(12): 1659-166

[55] Drake C, Roehrs T, Shambroom J, Roth, T. 2013. Caffeine Effects on Sleep Taken 0,3, or 6 hours before going to bed. Journal of Clinical Sleep Medicine. http://dx.doi.org/10.5664/jcsm.3170).

[56] Jaehne A, Loessl B, Barkai Z, Riemann D, Hornyak M. Effects of nicotine on sleep during consumption, withdrawal, and replacement therapy. Sleep Med Rev. 2009;13(5):363-377.

Caviness M, Anderson, B, Stein, M. Impact of Nicotine and Other stimulants on Sleep in Young Adults. Journal of Addiction Med. 2019;13(3):209-214)

[57] Hauri, P, Shirley, L.*No More Sleepless Nights*. New York City, NY. John Wiley &Sons; 1996

[58] Adapted from "7 Strategies for Serene Sleep." Arizona Integrative Medicine Fellowship Syllabus, 2014.

MOVE

[59] Olshansky, S., Al., E., Preston, S., Baker, M. G., Boulware, D. R., & Cavalcanti, A. B.,et al. (2005). A potential decline in life expectancy in the United States in the 21st century: *NEJM.*

[60] Standford Healthcare. Osteoporotic Fractures. (2019, December).   https://stanfordhealthcare.org/medical-conditions/back-neck-and-spine/osteoporotic-fractures.html

[61] O Barbosa Barreto de Brito, L., Rabelo Ricardo, D., Sardinha Mendes Soares de Arau´jo, D., Santos Ramo, P., Myers, J., & Gil Soares de Arau´jo, C. (2012). Ability to sit and rise from the floor as a predictor of all-cause mortality. *European Journal of Preventive Cardiology.*

BREATHE

[62] Meditation in Depth. National Center for Complimentary and Integrative Medicine.
https://www.nccih.nih.gov/health/meditation-in-depth.
April 2014.

[63] Rakel, D. *Integrative Medicine 4th Edition.* Philadelphia, PA: Elsevier; 2017.

[64] Briggs, J. (2010) Letter from the Director NCCIH, National Center for Complimentary and Integrative Medicine.
https://www.nccih.nih.gov.

[65] Kabat-Zinn, J. An outpatient Program in behavrioral medicine for chronic pain patients based on the practice of mindfulness meditation: theoretical considerations and preliminary results. *General Hospital Psychiatry*.1982; 4(1): 33-47.

[66] Luders E, Kurth F, Mayer EA, et al. The unique brain anatomy of meditation practitioners: alterations in cortical gyrification. *Frontiers in Human Neuroscience*. 2012;6:1–9.

[67] Luders E. Exploring age-related brain degeneration in meditation practitioners. *Annals of the New York Academy of Sciences*. 2013;1307:82–88.

[68] Desbordes G, Negi LT, Pace TW, et al. Effects of mindful-attention and compassion meditation training on amygdala response to emotional stimuli in an ordinary, non-meditative state. *Frontiers in Human Neuroscience*. 2012;6:1–15.

[69] Goyal M, Singh S, Sibinga EM, et al. Meditation programs for psychological stress and well-being: a systematic review and meta-analysis. *JAMA Internal Medicine*. 2014;174(3):357–368.

[70] Chen KW, Berger CC, Manheimer E, et al. Meditative therapies for reducing anxiety: a systematic review and meta-analysis of randomized controlled trials. *Depression and Anxiety*. 2012;29(7):545–562

[71] Clarke TC, Barnes PM, Black LI, Stussman BJ, Nahin RL. Use of yoga, meditation, and chiropractors among U.S. adults aged 18 and older. NCHS Data Brief, no 325. Hyattsville, MD: National Center for Health Statistics. 2018.

[72] Rakel, D. Integrative Medicine 4th Edition. Philadelphia, PA: Elsevier;2017

[73] Kabat-Zinn, J. (2014) *Mindfulness meditation in everyday life and exercises and meditations*. Better Listen Audio Produc-tion.

Audiobook and website, Greater Good in Action: Science-based practices for a Meaningful Life (Walking Meditation. Greater Good Science Center at UC Berk-ley and Hope Lab. https://ggia.berkeley.edu/prac-tice/walking_medita-tion)

Additional Reference

Blood Pressure

Alexander, R., Schneider, F. Staggers, et al. (1996) Trial of stress reduction for hypertension in older African Ameri-cans. *Hypertension.* 228-237 1996 8707387

Brook, R. D., Appel, R. J., & Rubenfire, M., et al. (2013). Beyond medications and diet: alternative ap-proaches to lowering blood pressure: a scientific state-ment from the American Heart Association. Hyperten-sion. 2013;61(6):1360–1383.

Gianfranco, A. S. (2004) Stress reduction and blood pres-sure control in hypertension: a role for transcen-dental med-itation? *J Hypertens.* 22:2057-2060 15480086